DOING FAMILY THERAPY

THE GUILFORD FAMILY THERAPY SERIES
Michael P. Nichols, Series Editor

Doing
Family Therapy

Second Edition

CRAFT AND CREATIVITY
IN CLINICAL PRACTICE

Robert Taibbi

THE GUILFORD PRESS
New York   London

To Susan

© 2007 The Guilford Press
A Division of Guilford Publications, Inc.
72 Spring Street, New York, NY 10012
www.guilford.com

Printed in the United States of America

This book is printed on acid-free paper.

Last digit is print number: 9 8 7 6 5 4 3 2 1

Library of Congress Cataloging-in-Publication Data

Taibbi, Robert.
    Doing family therapy: craft and creativity in clinical practice /
Robert Taibbi. — 2nd ed.
        p. ; cm. — (The Guilford family therapy series)
    Includes bibliographical references and index.
    ISBN-13: 978-1-59385-478-2 (hardcover: alk. paper)
    ISBN-10: 1-59385-478-1 (hardcover: alk. paper)
    ISBN-13: 978-1-59385-477-5 (pbk.: alk. paper)
    ISBN-10: 1-59385-477-3 (pbk.: alk. paper)
    1. Family therapy. I. Title. II. Series.
    [DNLM: 1. Family Therapy—methods. WM 430.5.F2 T129d
2007]
    RC488.5.T33 2007
    616.89′156—dc22
                                                    2007005098

Preface

The process of writing a new edition of a book, especially after more than 10 years, is a bit like digging up old photos of yourself, or stumbling upon long-past journal entries detailing the latest excitements and woes in your life at that moment. It's an opportunity not only to reflect on how much you and your life have changed over the years, but sometimes to be reassured just how much has remained the same.

Such has been the case with writing this new edition. Over a decade my values and assumptions have managed to stay intact, though a few appear to have hardened. The new edition's expanded section on sources of resistance, for example, seems to be a stronger statement of what I had begun to feel a decade ago, and goes hand in hand with my renewed belief that people are always doing their best. Some ideas on which I spend more space here are simply ones that I've grown more fond of and found increasingly useful in practice—the notion, for example, that many problems are really bad solutions to other, deeper problems—as a starting point for helping clients become curious about the problems in their lives. Other ideas reflect greater clarity in my clinical thinking that has emerged from my teaching and clinical practice—the list of the six most common family structures, for example, or the more detailed guidelines for helping parents manage the emotionality of their teenagers.

The changes in the field itself over the past decade have also seeped into my thinking. We've seen a shift, particularly in the community mental health movement, from the principles of client-centered services to client-directed services to the current notion of consumer-driven services, reflecting the growing belief in the power of the client as an active participant and partner in his or her own treatment. While there is increased reliance on medication, even with young children, there is also interest in and application of new alternatives—mindfulness and energy therapies, for example—as valuable supplements to traditional approaches. The research on brain chemistry, and particularly the studies of the impact of trauma on brain physiology, have substantially changed how we look at the source of and solutions to behavioral difficulties, and have given us a better idea of what really works when therapy works. And finally there has been the continuing presence of managed care with its focus on the individual, its concern with individual diagnosis, and its emphasis on limited treatment and medication, all of which was only just beginning 10 years ago. The forces of managed care have pushed most of us to think in terms of shorter-term treatment models, as well as made us all more sensitive to documentation, medical record audits, and liability issues. Some of this reshaping is reflected in my expanded discussions of ethical issues, my inclusion of a larger discussion on the role of touch in therapy, and my stronger encouragement to lean on supervisors as a resource.

The broader mental health field's increased focus on individual biology, diagnosis, and case management would seem to push traditional family therapy to a back burner. Yet I believe these changes have simply deepened and even expanded family therapy's paradigm and purpose. I've always seen family therapy's original mission as fairly straightforward—namely, that by creating healthier family systems we create healthier family members, a way of the many healing each other. Now we recognize a new challenge and opportunity—discovering ways that the family group, the many, can help heal an individual member who may be suffering from a loss or a disorder.

What I noticed most in the rewriting itself was a subtle shift in language, specifically substituting "helping" clients for "telling" clients. There's less of a directive, militant style in my work these days. I'm truly more the facilitator; this stance has the advantage, I believe, of seeing the larger picture of a family's circumstances simply because I am outside of them. I also found myself talking more and more about process, and particularly the process in the room—a reminder not only to the reader but to myself of the limits of my power and its focus.

The initial theses of the original book—that there are multiple approaches to most problems; that good therapy is *your* good therapy, a mix of your own personality and skills, your unique perspectives, values, and theoretical frameworks; that good therapy, like life, is pragmatic and practical—still constitute the strong core of this edition. What has been added to this is my deeper appreciation for the power of telling and listening. I never fail to be startled by the way people are changed simply by putting their stories into words, by having these stories deeply listened to, and by hearing the stories with which others respond. This, of course, is the primal foundation to relationships and healing that we've known all along, but it's good to realize that its power remains.

My thanks to all who have used this book over the past years, to the students and new clinicians who have passed along to me their kind comments and suggestions, to the people I've met on the road and through e-mails who have taken the time to tell me what they liked. I am grateful that I have had this opportunity to write, be read, and reflect.

About the Author

Robert Taibbi, LCSW, has over 34 years of experience primarily in community mental health as a clinician, supervisor, and clinical director. He is the author of *Clinical Supervision: A Four-Stage Process of Growth and Discovery*, several book chapters, and over 150 journal and magazine articles. He has served as teen advice columnist for *Current Health* and as a contributing editor to *Your Health and Fitness*, and has received two national writing awards for Best Consumer Health Writing from the National Health Information Resource Center.

Mr. Taibbi provides training nationally in family therapy, treatment of emotionally disturbed children and adolescents, and clinical supervision. He is currently in private practice in Charlottesville, Virginia.

Contents

Contents

[1]

Family Therapy

WELCOME TO OZ

They shuffle into your office without saying a word—first appointment and nobody is happy. The six-year-old boy immediately goes for your desk chair; the mother, a large woman in a faded green dress, nails him before he can hit the seat—"A.J., that's the lady's seat. Come sit over here." She rocks back and forth on the chair without standing up and stretches out one of her massive arms toward him; her tone is moderately firm. A.J. hesitates for a moment, then shrugs his shoulders and sits next to her with his head down. She reaches over and rubs his back.

The father is sitting across the room from the mother, and he has pulled his chair back so that it's almost in the corner. In contrast to his wife, he's as thin as one of the chair legs. He looks like he just got off work. His work boots still have mud on them, his uniform looks dusty. The name on the pocket says Ed. He doesn't look up at you, but surveys his fingers, then begins to pick at some dirt under one of his nails.

Next to you is the daughter, a blond-haired, attractive girl, thirteen, maybe fourteen. She's chewing gum and jiggling her foot, looking straight ahead, staring, it seems, at the molding behind the couch.

"So," you say, "thanks for coming. Glad to see you were all able to make it." You smile and try to make eye contact with everyone in the room. No one meets your eyes except for the mother, who is now sitting at the edge of her seat.

"Momma, I gotta go to the bathroom." A.J. tugs on his mother's sleeve and wiggles in his chair. The mother takes a quick glance at him, raises her index finger to her lips, and pats his knee.

"Momma, I gotta go now."

"A.J., sit still!" You're startled by the loud thud of a command from the father who is now staring at his son.

A.J. ignores him. "Momma, Momma." His voice is getting whiny; he's tugging at his mother's sleeve again and has shifted from wiggling to bouncing up and down on the seat.

"Now, you can just wait a few minutes, A.J., while we talk to this lady." The mother's voice has that strained sweet tone to it; she reaches over and starts rubbing his back again.

"Damn it, Lynn, why didn't you get him to go before we came?"

Time to get to work. "Ed, it seems—"

"Because he didn't need to, that's why." Lynn glares and stretches out her neck and words at the same time toward her husband. Then she turns back to A.J., and her voice shifts back to its saccharine tone, "Go ahead, honey, if you need to go. Just ask the lady if it's all right."

"He can wait!" Ed slams both hands down on the arm of the chair.

"Momma—"

"A.J., shut up!" Ed hooks his hands around the chair arms, threatening to get up.

You try again. "Ed, how—"

"The boy's got to go, Ed!"

"Hold it, everybody," you say, raising your voice. Things are starting to get out of control.

"Listen, you're the one who dragged me down here to talk to some stranger," says Ed, flicking his hand toward you, "all because of your precious little boy who—"

"Well, Ed, I sure as hell don't want him to turn out like you!" Lynn is now screaming, waving her arm. "Like you, Ed!"

"Momma, I got—"

"Okay, everybody," you croak, "let's—"

"I swear I don't need this!" Ed stands up and kicks the chair back against the wall. "And I don't need you, bitch." In a flash he swings the door open, stomps out and slams it shut.

"Momma, I got to go."

The daughter keeps staring at the molding.

SWEPT AWAY

This, of course, is one of the family therapist's worst nightmares. The family that breaks out the guns and knives before you even get the fee set. The family that stages a mutiny and gangs up on you—"Do *you* have children?" "Are you telling me that I should let him run around 'til three in the morning?" "We tried being nice, we tried being tough, but it doesn't help." "You don't understand, young lady, I have bad nerves." And worst of all, perhaps, the family that just won't talk.

Individual therapy always seems easier. One on one, no distractions, the quiet intimacy of the therapeutic relationship. As you listen deeply, soaking in both what is said and not said, the client's internal world, layer by layer, slowly unfolds. The vulnerable and fearful are named and by naming are known.

Family therapy is a different world all together. Like Dorothy, you're swept up and suddenly dropped down into a realm that seems strange, bewildering, intimidating. Even though it's your office, you're the outsider. Six people talking at once, each wanting your attention, each testing the limits ("Psst, Johnny, hand me that basketball"; "I want to go to the bathroom"; "Can I go get a Coke from the machine?"), everyone talking at once, blaming someone else or waiting for you to blame them, wanting you to tell them what to do to fix the problem five minutes after they sit down. A group of people with their own history and culture and language. Secret signals—the biting of a lip, a quiet laugh, the shaking of a head, the clenching of a fist—that suggest pools of stored resentments, private grudges, painful conflicts touched off by the most innocent of questions; a chain reaction that can spiral out of control before you have a chance to glance up from your notes or catch your breath.

That is how it seems to go in family therapy—too much happens too fast. You're less of a guide and more of a referee. The sigh that hung in the air and seemed so poignant in individual therapy is now quickly swallowed up by the stepfather's smirk. The intimate conversation between the caring but frightened mother and her lonely and awkward adolescent daughter suddenly dissolves when the four-year-old decides she can't handle it and insists that she going to throw up right there and then.

And then there are the stories—he said . . . , she said . . . , they said . . . —today, last Friday, 30 years ago. Stories of the past, stories about people long dead yet strangely alive and powerful, stories of hurt, stories that show just how bad things can get or how good they can possibly be. The heap of facts, figures, and perspectives from all corners of the room that can quickly drown the best family therapist, if he or she is not careful.

Yes, family therapy can be tough. It requires a flexibility, a creativity, and a willingness to approach your anxiety and at times to fly by the seat of your pants.

What can make this all the more difficult, especially for those new to the field, is the bewildering array of approaches from which to choose. Over the years traditional family therapy approaches—structural, strategic, narrative, multisystemic, wraparound, solution-focused—have morphed and been reshaped by changes in the workplace, culture, and larger therapy field. Managed care; client-directed treatment; best-practice home-based models; the growing sensitivity to the impact of multiculturalism, racism, sexuality, class, and developmental issues have had their impact and increased the number of perspectives available to the family therapist. The increasing array of techniques—from energy therapies such as EMDR (eye movement desensitization and reprocessing) to new behavioral approaches—have added to the therapists' array of tools. And, of course, the increase in the role of medication and the influence of our growing knowledge of the workings of the brain have made family therapy no longer a one-size-fits-all approach.

How do you decide which of these techniques and approaches are best to incorporate into your practice—for you, for your client family—when they all claim to be right or important? How do you not only keep track of all the things going on in the room, but at the same time also keep track of what is going on inside your head? How do you keep from feeling overwhelmed when you already feel overwhelmed? Why bother with it all? Why not just keep it simple, you think. Go ahead and just see Mrs. Jones by herself and leave Tommy to the guidance counselor at school.

Today there is a such a bewildering variety of new approaches, each with its own specialized approach to treatment, that it often seems impossible to keep up or to find a solid footing to stand upon. But it is there, in the form of basic family therapy concepts: that problems that seem to reside within one person actually involve the entire system; that the family not only unwittingly helps maintain the problem, but can serve as the resource for resolving it; that our job is less about telling them who is right and wrong, and more about helping them see how the patterns they created are no longer effective, that they can learn together new, more functional ways of interacting.

These practical, basic ideas, together with specific family therapy techniques, form the heart of the family therapy approach. Like the ballast on a ship, they can keep you steady when you begin to lose your balance in the swirl of a family session. They are the anchor that can keep you grounded whenever you begin to feel overwhelmed. One of the goals of this book is to familiarize you with these concepts and tools.

But the other goal of this book is to go beyond survival—to help you not only get through your sessions, but do it well, so that both you and the family can feel successful. This means worrying less about following the chapter and verse of a particular theory and drawing instead upon your own creativity and flexibility. This is the key to good family therapy—drawing upon and utilizing all your strengths, style, and values. Working with families in this way not only helps your clients by giving them most of what you have to offer, namely, more of yourself, but in the long run keeps you energized and sane.

Developing a creative and personally unique approach to family therapy is different from what is often the common end product of formal education and the learning process. Rather than feeling encouraged to discover themselves, new therapists often wind up only imitating others or feeling pressured to choose an allegiance to a certain school or theory—you become a structuralist, an object relations person, a staunch believer in cognitive-behavioral approaches. Rather than styling your approach around your values and strengths, you squeeze yourself into an a particular model; you not only feel constricted, but are forced to leave important parts of yourself out. Gradually, to no one's surprise, you become what you present yourself as, and left-out parts of your personality are forgotten or become dormant.

If staying anchored means learning to rely on a basic core of concepts, staying creative means realizing that there isn't only one approach to any family. This is the pragmatic, individualized approach to family therapy that we'll be focusing on together. Through case examples we'll look at options—the multiple ways of tackling a family and their concerns—so that you can learn to map out alternative routes that not only fit your skills and the family's resources, but can keep you both moving when a particular path seems blocked.

This book is divided into three parts. In the first section we map out the terrain of family therapy, the basic skills that keep you afloat, the obstacles and dangers, and the ways to handle them in the beginning, middle, and end stages of treatment.

In the second section we look at a variety of cases and problems. Here's where we talk about applying the basic skills, exploring clinical options, and sorting out your own preferences and style. Through this process you'll learn to think creatively and make use of your intuitions.

Finally, in the third section, we return to some practical tips for dealing with the pressures of the work, especially in agency settings, ways of staying emotionally healthy over the long haul, and managing the daily wear and tear of the work. We also step back and explore work in the larger context of your everyday living, the role of work and therapy in light of your beliefs and values, what it means to have a calling, and what it takes to have integrity.

Along the way there are exercises for you to try that can help you see how the concepts of the chapter may apply to your personal and professional life. These give you a chance to further define your strengths, skills, and values.

But before we begin this exploration we need to talk a bit about the basic ingredients that are the starting points for becoming a good family therapist.

[2]

Of Theory, Philosophy, and Courage

THEORY—SOMETHING TO HOLD ONTO

An effective therapist needs to be grounded in some kind of theory. Too many theories can overwhelm you, the wrong kind can constrict you, but have none and you are set adrift in a vast ocean of facts and observations. A theory of therapy gives you something to hold onto. It can be as simple or complex as you like, because what a theory says is less important than what it can give to you and allow you to do.

Theories fulfill several important functions. First they are, by definition, tools for organizing. They are the Peg-Board upon which we hang what we see and hear; they show us where to look and what to listen for. Events that once seemed random are now seen as connected. A father's hunting trip with his son is no longer just a family folktale but, when hung on the theory, becomes an example of role modeling, an attempt to resolve and repair some split from the past, or yet another way of avoiding growing tension within the marriage. A daughter's unexpected running away from home is not the ridiculous ending to a stupid argument about shoes, but an understandable, even predictable way of coping with undisclosed sexual abuse, a response to the father's life-draining depression, or part and parcel of the larger cycle of addiction. With your theory as a lens, behavior and words suddenly have meaning and merit. Seemingly unrelated events and reactions are now linked to a larger family process, a deeper layer of problems that not only explain what has happened, but tell what can happen in the future. Most importantly, your theory can provide a road map for changing it.

With the organization that theory provides comes an increase in your personal sense of control. Think back to your first interviews with families, couples, or even individuals. In the middle of it you probably felt swamped by the tidal wave of facts and emotions coming at you, and no doubt left the session bleary-eyed and exhausted. With the theory's ability to help us bundle facts together and dismiss others entirely, anxiety that potentially can make us ineffective is reduced. When we fear becoming overwhelmed in the process of the session—by the conflicting stories about what happened last Thursday, the building emotions of Dad's anger or Mom's sadness—we can lean on our theory to tell us what to ask or do to gather the information we need. As we read the intake sheet we use our theory to help us start filling in the blanks, formulating a hypothesis that we can take into the initial session with us. The theory becomes then, not only a tool but a support, an internal security blanket, something we can always return to. With it we have courage to walk into the unfamiliar world of the family; we feel prepared, rather than confused and apprehensive.

But theory not only helps you, it helps your clients as well. Through the filter of your theory old behaviors are suddenly seen with new eyes. Neutral words replace those laden with anger and blame: "I can understand, Ms. Smith, why you are feeling frustrated, but Davon isn't just trying to give you a hard time; he is hyperactive and it is harder for him to sit still than it is for Shameka"; "Did you all see what just happened?—Mom, you made a suggestion, Dad, you disagreed, you both start to argue, and Mary whines as a way to distract you and get you to stop. This pattern is one that you all easily fall into. Patterns can automatically sweep you up. Every family has patterns; this is one of yours."

By seeing their problem in such a new light, by "reframing" the problem, by talking to themselves with different words, the family discovers ways out of the psychological and emotional mental ruts in which they were constantly spinning. New, more creative solutions become possible—Johnny isn't a bad kid who needs to be punished, but has a biochemical disorder that makes it hard for him to do certain things; I'm not really going crazy, I just need to talk to someone about my sadness; our relationship isn't lousy simply because we're both stubborn, but because our needs over the years have changed. The theory opens new doors to the solving of problems, the process of healing.

While all theories are by definition useful for organizing, naming, and supporting, the one you choose as your template in your everyday work should be the one that fits you the best. This means that you shouldn't settle on a particular theory just because it's what you were exposed to in school. You shouldn't choose one because it intellectually appeals to you, is popular with your colleagues, or even seems to work with certain problems. The best theory for you is the theory that meets you halfway. It should fit your personality, strengths, and personal philosophy—your assumptions, values, and notions of what life is and the role people and problems play in it. When there's that kind of a match, a close fitting of the basic you and the theory you embrace, it supports you rather than you supporting it. It underscores your natural instincts and intuitions. Rather than feeling constricted or constrained, you feel empowered.[1]

interesting

what is my personality?

How does one distinguish this

PHILOSOPHY—LOOKING AT THE BIGGER PICTURE

So, what is your personal philosophy? What do you believe?

Honestly answering these questions takes some time and reflection. All too many of us don't take the time to figure it out, don't know the right questions to ask ourselves, or don't have the words to articulate what we feel. Rather than doing the hard work of doing our own discovering and defining, we're often inclined to take the shorter path and grab on to what's already in front of us, namely, the personal philosophies of others—our parents, friends, spouses, or those we read in books or learn in class.

This works fine until it doesn't work, and eventually it doesn't work. We're adapting ourselves to something that's made for someone else, and at some point there's a strain—who we are and how we live grow ever wider apart. We feel bored or empty, we have a "crisis" in our career, in our lives. Nothing seems right, something seems to be missing, we itch for change, but don't really know what we want to change.

This is particularly true, I believe, for many clinicians. In my own

[1] A good place to start your search for theory, I believe, is in old and new family therapy classics. Look at Murray Bowen, *Family Therapy in Clinical Practice*, Jason Aronson, 1994; Salvador Minuchin, *Families and Family Therapy*, Harvard University Press, 1974; Jay Haley, *The Art of Strategic Therapy*, Brunner-Routledge, 2003; Michael White, *Narrative Means to Therapeutic Ends*, Norton, 1990; David Scharff *Object Relations Family Therapy*, Jason Aronson, 1991; Scott Miller et al., *Handbook of Solution-Focused Brief Therapy*, Jossey-Bass, 1996.

personal life and in my experience with new therapists over the years, I've found that many who go into the helping professions were most often "good kids" as children. Being good, meeting expectations, being sensitive to the needs and emotions of the bigger and stronger parents are ways a child can cope in the world of adults, and quickly the child learns that he or she can get positive attention for this way of being. Essentially, the stance the good kid adapts is one of "If they're happy, I'm happy, and I need to make sure they are happy." As an adult this learned sensitivity to others becomes the foundation for empathy; helping others be happy becomes the initial drive to enter the therapy field.

But there's a downside to this. With the focus always outward, always toward others, the good kid often fails to learn what he or she really wants. Instead, his or her mind is filled with "shoulds," the rules and expectations of others. Knowing what you want only comes from exploration, that is, stepping away from the rules and taking risks. What usually emerges first is not what you want, but an awareness of what you don't want, don't like, no longer believe—what you may be ready to give up.

This elimination process of finding out what you don't like helps you eventually define what you do like; it sets the cornerstone of personal empowerment and creativity. What enabled Dorothy to survive in the strange Land of Oz—to make the tough decisions and find courage—was not only her memory of home, but the philosophy and values of home. In the face of great outer challenges she pushed against her own grain, and rediscovered what was most important to her. You too need to do the same, that is, rediscover what you truly know and believe, name the values that run your life. When you hear the philosophies and theories of the families in your office, or read about them in books by fellow clinicians, measure them against your own and see what doesn't fit, what you don't agree with as well as what you do. From your reactions and introspection you can craft your own life philosophy, and use it as a starting point for identifying the theories that support it.

When you feel disillusioned by the grind of the work, pessimistic about your ability to help, or burned out by simple wear and tear, you can go back to your philosophy to reignite your creativity. Just as our theory helps us fill in the holes in our clinical understanding and points the direction we need to go, our personal philosophy helps us fill in the holes during our times of confusion and doubt, and points us back to what we know is right for us. Our personal philosophy not only gives us a running summary of what we believe, but a continual vision of what we can become.

Here are some questions to help you recognize what you know and believe:

What is the most important thing in life? (Trust the first thing that comes to your mind.)

What is the purpose of life? What is the purpose of *your* life? What can only you give, create, do?

What is the meaning of relationships, of families? What is our responsibility toward others?

Why do relationships change? How much can people change? How do we know when change is necessary?

What are the limits of relationships? When should relationships end? What does commitment mean?

What is the relationship between doing for yourself and doing for others?

What does it mean to love someone or something?

What should parents most teach their children? What are the limits of the parents' responsibility, involvement?

What is the role of emotions in our lives?

What is the purpose of work?

How much of our life is controlled by our past?

Big questions that you may or may not have ready answers to. As you think about them, other questions may come to mind, or you may realize that your ideas have been taken in whole from others and may benefit from your own further scrutiny. It's not the content of the questions themselves that are important so much as the questioning process itself.[2]

COURAGE

Theory and philosophy together create a foundation upon which skills develop; the mix of all three—theory, philosophy, skills—form the nucleus of good therapy. But there is limit to how much theory and philosophy can support us, how far skills can carry us. The final ingredient that the good clinician needs is courage.

[2]Another book that may expand your thinking on philosophy further is George Simon, *Beyond Technique in Family Therapy*, Allyn & Bacon, 2002.

Few of us would list therapy up there among the world's most danger-ous professions—there are no high-speed chases, ducking of bullets, bal-ancing on the edge of rooftops, or handling of dangerous heavy machin-ery. Instead we sit around on blue couches or wingback chairs, sipping coffee, asking how the past week went, looking reflective, occasionally furrowing a brow or patting a client on the shoulder—hardly the stuff of drama and danger. But the inner journey can be just as perilous as the outer, and risk, and the courage needed to face it, is required nonetheless. Courage, after all, comes from dealing with the fear and anxiety that lie inside, no matter what the source.

This anxiety and fear are powerful. It's no surprise, perhaps, that cli-ents often talk about feeling as though they are perched at the edge of cliff or that there is bomb inside them ready to explode—their sense of per-sonal danger is absolutely accurate. It's fear, after all, not foolishness or ig-norance, that usually keeps our lives stuck and stagnant. In families it's the interlocking of each family member's fears that compounds upon itself to make any change ever more difficult. Your success and failure as a ther-apist come less from knowing what to do, and more from pushing hard enough to propel the family members out of the constraints that they nat-urally place around their lives. Your most basic of goals is helping steer people through the anxiety of change, teaching and showing them that if they stick it out and get through that minefield of fear about the un-known, that good things can be found on the other side.

It starts with you. You are the role model and the coach. You, as the outsider, are the one who can see what in new directions the family needs to go or can go and can guide them toward it. This doesn't mean taking foolish chances, but it does mean having the courage to move against the family's natural inertia, to raise the thorny issues that no one wants to talk about, much less change. This means confronting the mother who ap-pears so fragile and makes others, including you, believe that she can't handle confrontation; talking to a child about the terrible things that happened to him or her without getting lost in your own grief and anger; or saying nothing at all so that the person across from you can finally say what he has been holding back for a long time. It means resisting the pres-sure you feel to fix people, take sides, make them change.

This is the everyday courage that doing therapy demands—pushing yourself to use your theory and skills creatively, mindfully. It's the courage of not only putting your own philosophy into practice, but of helping others to define, refine, and eventually live theirs. It's the simple courage of honesty and approaching challenges and anxiety rather than avoiding it. It's acknowledging both the gift of seeing much of your own life in the life of others and the danger of becoming confused over who you are trying to help. It is the willingness to try something in order to move ahead, even if you aren't exactly sure where it will lead.

Good therapy requires control, but is not controlling; constantly facing the unpredictable while just as constantly predicting that the unpredictable will come; fostering intimacy while keeping clear limits on that intimacy; being committed but being willing to stop when it seems an end has been reached or will never come. Good therapy is a seeming hodgepodge of contradictions and qualifiers that requires that you walk a thin line between too little and too much, between reaching out and holding back. Courage is the stuff that glues the contradictions together, keeps you steady on the line, gets you moving until skill, knowledge, and self-trust can take over. Without it the families you see are penned in, confined to the narrow range of your own comfort; with it they can begin to experience their lives in the new way.

These three, then—theory, philosophy, and courage—are the prerequisites for journeying through the Land of Oz that is family therapy. We'll be talking more about them as we explore the technical aspects of treatment and discuss specific case examples. Keep them in mind as you move through this information. In the next chapter we review some basic family therapy concepts.

Looking Within: Chapter 2 Exercises

At the end of each chapter throughout this book you will find a number of exercises and questions designed to make the material in the chapter more personally relevant, to ground the concepts within your own practice.

It may be tempting to just read these and not actually do them. Try not to. If, after starting, an exercise seems too redundant or irrelevant, go ahead and move on to the next. But if the exercise stirs your curiosity or, better yet, your anxiety, give it a try. You have nothing to lose, and you may be surprised at what you find.

1. A short imagery exercise: Go to a quiet place for a few minutes where you know you won't be disturbed. Sit comfortably in your chair. Take a few deep breaths, and for a few moments just concentrate on your breathing. Begin to feel relaxed.

   See if you can see in your mind's eye a meadow. It is a bright, warm, sunny day; the grass is green, flowers are in bloom and the air smells sweet with their fragrance, a slight breeze blows. And there you see yourself, walking along, feeling relaxed, the sun warm on your back. As you are walking, you see ahead of you the edge of a wood. You decide to walk toward it.

   As you approach the woods, you begin to hear in the breeze the sound of a name, the name of a person of the same sex as you. As you near the edge of the wood and peer into the darkness of the trees you are aware that someone is there in the shadows, the person whose name you heard. You become curious; you begin to wonder who this person is, what he or she is like. Then you listen and can tell that this person is coming toward you.

   A person emerges from the trees. Notice how he or she looks. Imagine yourself starting a conversation with this person. Imagine asking all the questions that you were curious about, finding out all you want to know that will tell you just what this person is like. Take as much time as you need talking to this person.

   When your conversation is over, the person waves good-bye and walks back into the wood. You turn around and begin to walk back down the meadow, thinking about all that you have just heard. When your fantasy feels over, just sit for a few minutes and relax.

   It is important to hold within ourselves (and help create for families) a vision of what we can be. This imagery exercise is designed to get you in touch with your ideal self. This may have been easy for you to do, or you may have had some difficulty. Perhaps you had sensations or recalled memories, or heard dialogue, but had trouble creating the images. Don't be concerned. You can try again another time, and will probably have a different response.

Be aware of the person you saw, not only his or her appearance, but of his or her personal qualities, his or her dreams, his or her attitudes toward others, toward life. Notice the gap between the way you see yourself now and the person you imagined. Is there anything that surprised you? Is there a particular quality that you most would like to develop? What would it take to do it?[3]

2. Look over once again the philosophical questions presented earlier. Try writing down the answers to as many as catch your interest. See if you can develop a short (a couple of sentences) concise personal statement of life, values, and work.

3. You don't need to take karate lessons or Outward Bound courses to increase your sense of courage. Simply begin by taking small risks, not just in your work, but elsewhere in your life. Practice approaching your fear—walk up to that neighbor on your block that you've seen a few time and start a conversation, ask a question in a group even though you know it sounds stupid, try something physically different even though you feel clumsy or know you're not good at it. Avoid telling lies for a couple of days and see what happens.

A half dozen times during the week, as you become aware of approaching the edges of your own anxiety, go forward, do whatever is scary, then pat yourself on the back. The goal is not to be without fear, but to be able to act in spite of it.

---

[3]This exercise was adapted from the work of Roberto Assagioli. See his *Psychosynthesis: A Collection of Basic Writing*, Synthesis Center, 2000, for additional imagery exercises.

[3]

Family Therapy
THE BASICS

A sk a couple to describe a typical argument—who starts the conversation, what happens next, how it escalates, how it ends—and without talking about any content, most can describe exactly what the pattern is, down to the slamming of the bedroom door, the "Go ahead, you're going to do what you want anyway!" retort, the getting in the car and driving off. As an experiment, try sitting in someone else's regular seat at the dinner table tonight and watch what happens. Just make sure the knives and guns are out of the house before you try it.

For all our talk about being our own person, in reality we spend most of our time engaged in never-ending ping-pong matches with others, where what we do and they do is always a series of set and predictable reactions to each other. With those to whom we are the closest—our family, our friends, our colleagues—knowing each other well means having each other's game moves down pat. We can see that slam argument coming 10 minutes before it arrives, sense out of the corner of our emotional eye the sarcastic remark that always zings past us before dropping off the edge of the conversation, know that his slight head fake to the right means he's about to cry. We can anticipate and respond to each other so reflexively that most of our interactions run completely on automatic pilot.

When this social volleying is compounded over and over with the people we interact with all day, we find our everyday lives filled with blocks of routine (morning wake-up/prework time, the work block, the dinnertime block, postdinner, and bedtime routine), handfuls of predictable social patterns ("Hi, how are you?"; "I'm fine"), and unspoken rules and deals that essentially are designed to merely keep the game going as it is ("You don't mention my drinking, and I won't mention your affair").

It would seem that these routines and rules are enough to flatten life, to make it deadly boring and uncreative, but, of course, they don't. On the contrary, it's precisely because of these predictable routines that we can run on remote for huge stretches of time and free up the mental and emotional energy within us that we need for innovative thinking, creative problem solving, and deliberate action. The slightest deviations in this regularity—the boss failing to respond to our "Good Morning" greeting, our partner forgetting our anniversary (or was it really forgetting?)—remind us that being creatures of habit keeps us from being perpetually anxious and insecure. All in all, it's the repetition and structure in our social world that save us the trouble of having to reinvent our lives each morning when we wake up.

But the downside of our dependency on routine and reaction is that these patterns can become unbelievably tenacious, our routines hard to break. As the dinnertable melee makes clear, any attempt to disrupt a pattern can wreak emotional havoc; the immediate reaction of the others is to pressure the rebel to fall back into line and keeping the pattern going.

It is this focus upon interactional patterns that is the basis of family therapy. In contrast to psychodynamic approaches whose perspective is more vertical and linear, seeing problems moving down into the individual and moving back in the past, family therapy's view is horizontal, kinetic, circular—focusing on the spaces between people, their round-robin of behaviors, the way the patterns are started and stopped as well as kept going. Families stay stuck because of the interlocking nature of repetitive interactions.

How you think shapes *what* you think you can and should do. Thinking in terms of circles and interpersonal connections, rather than lines and individual pasts, changes the shape of therapy. If the patterns are circular, then where you start isn't all that important since circles are notorious for not having starting points. If everything is interconnected; then whether you talk to the parents then see the child, or see the child and then the parents, work on the marriage or help the parents set up some structure theoretically doesn't make any difference—the pieces and the parts and the patterns will all eventually emerge as you look for them and gather them together. What is important is that the pattern change, because it is the pattern that holds the problem. Whether you do this with the entire family, including the dog, or just the most motivated person of the group doesn't theoretically matter because if even only one person is able to stick to his or her guns (think Gandhi or Martin Luther King here), the pattern is broken and will, with persistence, eventually collapse.

This view makes change valuable for itself; the act of change, moving against one's grain and habit, can start the chain reaction that can break apart the patterns in which the problems and emotions are suspended. Precisely what the change is or where it is often is less important than the presence of some type of change.

What is wonderful and freeing about this way of thinking is that there is less need to worry about doing it "right." It's easy when seeing an experienced colleague in action or, worse yet, to see one of the masters—Salvador Minuchin, Insoo Berg, Jay Haley, Virginia Satir, Carl Whitaker, Michael White—at work on tape or in person to feel that he or she has figured it all out, has made that perfect match between the particular problem and the proper solution. So you carefully watch his or her every move, transcribe word for word his or her response, practice getting just the right inflection in your voice, asking the questions in just the right order. In your mind you keep a running chart of problems and their matching strategies. If you can just do what they do, think how they think, you too, you feel, can be, if not a master therapist, at least competent.

But no matter how effective they seem, their way is not the only way. The basic goals that power family therapy are less delicate and precise than what may appear through the work of the experts; the intent is more broad, more general—to stop the patterns, or make the family aware of the patterns so they can stop them themselves and create brand new ones. The good family therapist is less a meticulous detective or brilliant strategist and more a shrewd and insightful anarchist, an unfailing resistance fighter.

This doesn't mean, of course, that as a family therapist you're left to bludgeon problems with only this blunt concept. You have at your disposal a range of techniques. It takes skill to choose those that better suit a particular problem and family, and sensitivity to help the family manage their anxiety as the dysfunctional patterns begin to come apart. What it does mean is that family systems theory gives you more room to move around. You have freedom to adjust what you do to best utilize your greatest strengths and the family's motivation. You can side step the battle with the client over where to start.

Finally, this way of thinking and working means you are not alone. Even though it seems that individual therapy offers you, as the clinician, greater control over the session process, this is more than offset by the presence of other family members in the room. They can add information and perspectives beyond what individual provides; they can demonstrate right before your eyes the dysfunctional patterns that are holding the problem in place.

MAPPING THE GROUND?— STARTING ASSUMPTIONS

Before looking more closely at the basics of family therapy, we need to look at the ground on which it's built, namely, some assumptions about therapy itself. Before beginning your clinical practice, it's valuable to be clear in your own mind about therapy's boundaries, bottom lines and givens; they'll form the outline of the map that you use in navigating through the work of family therapy. Your answers to some of the questions raised in the last chapter may have revealed to you many of your assumptions. The following are mine—once again, measure them against your own:

• *Therapy is one option among many for creating change and solving problems.* I once worked with a woman individually who was struggling with a number of problems in her marriage. She became aware of some of the dynamics, was able to change some of the patterns within the relationship itself, but for every step forward she felt she was taking two back. Depression set in. We discussed hospitalization because her symptoms were getting steadily worse. Then one Monday she came for her appointment totally different. She felt great, much less anxious and depressed. She had a much clearer sense of what she wanted and was willing to do even, though she hadn't made any drastic changes in her relationship. She had had a life-changing experience.

Over the weekend, she explained, as she was lying on the couch feeling miserable and hopeless, she found herself actually contemplating suicide, imaging going upstairs, getting sleeping pills from the bathroom, taking the bottle, lying back down on the couch where she would fall forever asleep. But even as these thoughts ran through her mind, others tied to her religious beliefs rose up as well. She remembered all the messages of all those childhood Sunday school classes; the power of God, the presence of Jesus always there to help, to love her. Suddenly she was overwhelmed by the sense of comfort and security; she felt that God was right there in the room at her side. She knew deep inside herself that everything would turn out all right if only she would recommit herself to life and love.

And so she did. This brief but powerful religious experience helped her to change, and even on follow-up a year later she was doing well. I've known other people over the years who have had just as powerful experiences: People who had come back from the brink of suicide by noticing a coworker smiling when she said "Good morning," or by simply writing with pencil and paper about their torment and life. People who joined a support group and after three meetings were already on the road to resolving a long-standing problem; people who found hope or inspiration in a magazine article or book, or in a casual, over-the-fence conversation with a neighbor; people who, without looking for change, found their view of life different simply by driving out West and looking up toward the sky from the bottom of a canyon.

It's all too easy for us as therapists to get tunnel vision, to feel evangelical about our work, and believe that folks need what only we can give them. But people have been solving problems and making changes for millennia without our help. Keeping that in mind helps us present what we have to offer more fairly and responsibly, helps prevent us from seeming arrogant or demanding, and reduces the pressure we may feel at times to provide the only salvation there is.

• *Therapy is a service.* There has been a gradual but dramatic evolution in the relationship between therapist and client in the past 60 years. In the heyday of psychoanalysis, therapy was wrapped in the aura and mystery of analysts who assumed they knew more than their patients but never revealed much about their thinking. Similarly, early family therapists assumed that only they understood clients' families, and they tended to be bossy and confrontive. In the past 10 or 15 years there has been a shift in the entire mental health field, first to "client-centered services," now to "consumer-driven services."[1]

---

[1]For more information about history of family therapy, see Michael Nichols and Richard Schwartz, *Family Therapy: Concepts and Methods*, Pearson, 2006.

These are amazing changes and reflect the servant/service model that has even infiltrated the leadership models of the business world. To say that I am offering you a service that is one among many open to you, a service that you can be an active participant in shaping means that the aura and one-up position of power is gone. Instead of clients coming in awe and in expectation of some psychological magic, they now come as consumers seeking, and paying for, for resources, information, advice, or coaching. We no longer "read minds," but instead are helpful because we have some specialized knowledge, because we are outside the individual and family system and therefore can see the blind spots that the family members themselves cannot see. Adopting this stance of service keeps us both humble and human, and it is through our humanity that clients can feel supported and understood.

This assumption also means that clients may come with different goals than what we have in mind. Many families, especially those who are referred to agencies, are crisis oriented—they are willing to come long enough to get what seems to be falling on their heads off, but may not be interested in coming longer to find out what caused it or see what they can do differently next time. Some will move beyond the presenting problem and explore some of the underlying dynamics but are not willing to move toward that place of empowerment or awareness that you, in your heart of hearts, wish for them. That's fine—it's their journey, and your role and commitment is only to help them as far as they are willing to go at this time.

But, you say, it's fine to talk about choices and service, but what about all those court-ordered cases, those families that obviously need to come but never would if not made to do so? We're back to values. I still say that I am offering a service that the family can choose to accept or not. If the court orders the counseling, the court is the one with the initial agenda, and I make that clear to the client. They still can come or not, and if not, I will be happy to tell the court, which can decide on the consequences. What the court is really interested in, I tell them, is not counseling as an end in itself, but rather change in some behavior that threatens the larger community—stopping abuse, going to school, stopping their drug use. If clients have another idea for solving the problem and changing their behavior, they have a right to try it because there are other options. Their challenge will be convincing the court that this other approach truly will work, and I may help them think that argument through.

If they decide to stay with me we will negotiate what we will work on. Since everything is connected, I'm not too concerned if the client doesn't immediately want to deal with the problem that the court wants him or her to deal with; I just don't want the client to waste my time coming simply for the sake of telling someone else that he or she showed up.

As a therapist I cannot foster intimacy or trust if my job is to be the enforcer. I prefer to leave that role to someone else.

• *People are always doing the best they can.* This follows naturally from the other two assumptions. What we see as problems are actually poor solutions to other, underlying problems. Think of addictions or cutting or eating disorders, or even abuse, where the parent either feels she is doing her best to correct a child, or has no other releases for managing the anger welling up inside. All these are poor solutions to deeper individual fears, anxieties, and angers. If you believe that people are doing the best they can in the moment, not only is it a more optimistic view of life, but then it is possible to be compassionate to others rather than taking the one-up judgmental stance. Your role no longer becomes one of uncovering their failings or correcting their mistakes, but helping them develop other means of coping. Rather than pretending to accept those copng methods you don't really like, you can honestly say, "I don't really understand, but I'd like to. Tell me more about it." Good therapy becomes less about fixing people and more about helping them become more flexible—to increase their range of emotions, perspectives, language, or behaviors—so they have more coping options, better solutions than the less successful, destructive, or limited ones that they currently employ.

Believing that people are always doing their best also essentially eliminates the notion of client resistance. I remember hearing Michael Trout, who does a lot of interesting work on attachment disorders, say once that when he first meets with a parent and a child he assumes, regardless of what happens in that session, that the parent is doing everything possible right then and there to help him understand exactly what the problem is and what they need. What a positive and empowering perspective this is, one so different from the notion of clients' "natural resistance" that fills so much of traditional therapeutic literature. If we believe people are doing their best, then the responsibility shifts to us to focus upon and repair what we might see as resistance or reluctance. In my way of thinking there are four basic sources of "resistance," all of which fall in the therapist's lap:

1. No agreed-upon problem: Some of this was touched upon earlier, but, in general, when there is a lack of clarity or disagreement (e.g., court vs. client) about what the problem, and hence the solution, is that we are focusing on.
2. Faulty expectations regarding the process: The client has different expectations about the therapist's role, the focus (e.g., see my child rather than the family), what occurs in a session (tell me what to do rather than ask a lot of questions), or the length of treatment (two sessions rather than two months)
3. Pacing: The clinician is moving too fast and the client is having trouble learning the skills, feels overwhelmed, and needs more support or information.
4. Replicating a family role: The therapist re-creates old roadblocks in the family process—for example, coming on too strong with a teen and being seen by the teen as much like his or her pushy father; the therapist works too hard to rescue the family and everyone becomes passive.[2]

We'll be discussing each of these in greater detail as we discuss skills and cases, but what's important to notice for now is that client resistance is not a given and not a mysterious process. If you believe that clients are doing the best they can, then their digging in of their heels is a sign that there is something askew in the room or in the relationship, and it's the responsibility of the therapist to figure it out and begin to correct it. After all, therapy is the clinician's world, not the client's, and the clinician is responsible for educating the client about the process and providing feedback and clarity about focus, goals, and expectations if they are to be on the same clinical page and achieve expected results.

The best of therapists needs to accept that he or she is incapable of controlling all the factors in the client's world that work against therapy, that not every client will be fully healed, and that through no particular fault of anyone, client or clinician, not every intake will ultimately result in completion of even modest goals. To expect otherwise is to put unrealistic pressure and expectations on ourselves and our clients. Other aspects of our lives are generally not so tidy and conclusive, and there is no reason

---

[2]A somewhat different but detailed and useful view of resistance can be found in Carol Anderson, *Mastering Resistance: A Practical Guide to Family Therapy*, Guilford Press, 1983.

to believe that therapy, which is only a more condensed form of life, can or should be much different.

• *The therapeutic relationship is important.* When I ask clients at termination what they remember most about their therapy, or, looking back, what they thought was most helpful, I'm always surprised how so many times it's not anything big and therapeutic that I thought I did that to them made a difference. It's usually the small things that were important—the two-second phone call when the client went into the hospital to see how he was feeling, the pat on the back on the way out after the third session, the way I played with the three-year-old, the story I told about my father's birthday as we were walking into my office, a follow-up letter after a missed appointment. These little gestures of humanity and concern become the glue that holds the relationship and therapy together; they convey to the client that here is respect, caring.

We learn this early on in Counseling 101, and it continues to remain true. Just as the little things can undo therapy, it's the little things that often keep it alive and make it valuable to the client, little things that come through the relationship itself. A therapy relationship has the potential to be a very different relationship than what the client is used to. It can be more committed or caring or confrontive than others in the client's life, and while this can be frightening for many, arousing old habits of distrust and avoidance, for many others it can be healing enough.

Most of all the therapeutic relationship has the potential simply to be more honest, where people say what they mean and mean what they say. Even if they change their mind and say something different five minutes later, the therapy session is the place where words match emotions and behavior matches thoughts. It's an honesty that begins with the clinician.

It's with these assumptions that I start family therapy. They form for me a framework around what I do; they help me stay clear about the limits and responsibilities of my power. Again, think about your own ideas about change; about your role and responsibility to the client, about the limits of your own power or the power of therapy to solve problems, and about the whole notion of client resistance and what should you do about it. Try to be as clear as possible about what you believe.

Looking Within: Chapter 3 Exercises

1. "Therapy is one option among many for creating change and solving problems." Do you believe that there are other approaches or methods that can be effective in helping others? What are they? Under what conditions might you suggest that a client consider such other options?

2. Under what conditions would you consider seeking therapy for yourself? What are your own reservations? What would you look for most in a therapist or in the process?

3. One of my assumptions is that people are always doing their best. Do you agree with this? What are your own assumptions about the basic nature of people?

4. What are your own thoughts about resistance in clients?

5. Therapeutic relationship versus therapeutic skill: While it could be argued that the ability to create a strong therapeutic relationship is a therapeutic skill, there is the notion (and research) that a strong relationship on its own can "make up for" a weaker technical arsenal. Do you agree with this? Are there particular problems or clients for which having specific skills would be most important?

[4]

The Basic Seven

Once your assumptions are clear the work can begin, and that work begins within your own mind. As you talk to the members of a family, as you gather information, as you watch how they behave while they are with you, begin to envision how this family can be different, how the family would look, sound, and operate if the problem that they grapple with most were not there, if the patterns that held their lives together were changed. It is this vision, this positive vision of what can be, that is the guiding light for the therapist, and when shared with the family, for them as well. It can empower them, point them in the right direction, and most of all give them hope.

But the vision-making process gets muddied when the family unravels problem after problem with no end in sight and shifts their burden directly onto your lap, when the family is paralyzed by powerful emotions which not only evaporate that new and fragile sense of promise, but paralyze you as well. Like tennis, piano playing, accounting, and baking, family therapy has its fundamentals, its basic concepts and skills. This core of ideas and skills is what you can always return to to recenter yourself and the family.

Recentering is the important word here. When I was studying meditation many years ago, I was taught to use a one-word mantra as my focus. The teacher stressed over and over that whenever I "caught" myself lost in meddlesome thoughts, I didn't need to feel concerned or guilty or worry about doing it right. I merely needed to stop and return back to the chant. In the beginning it was easy to wander off into the forest of my own plans and worries—the argument I had had with my wife that morning, the list of items I needed to get at the hardware store, the upcoming deadline on the report at work—without even being aware of it. It seemed that I was returning to the mantra more than I was actually saying it. But with practice this changed—I was more and more able to stay with the mantra before wandering off.

So it is with family therapy. When you find yourself lost in the family, overwhelmed by their words, their questions, their emotions, don't panic and don't kick yourself for messing up. Simply keep in mind these basic skills for navigating the process, and get recentered. In the beginning you may find yourself seemingly always going back, but with practice your forays into the thick of the family will go increasingly farther. Even with a lot of experience, you'll sometime get overloaded, and it's good to know you can always go back and start again.

What follows are family therapy basics. Each of these is one vital part of the foundation; together they interlock to form the backbone of both systems theory and good family therapy. Keeping these seven basic practices in mind can help you stay on track through the most difficult sessions. Once you feel comfortable with them you can use them as the basis for improvisation. Mix and match these the way a good chef mix and matches his or her favorite ingredients to create your own style, your own unique approach to a particular problem or family. In the first section of this book we map them out; in the second section we talk more about the creative variations.

1. DETERMINE WHAT IS THE PROBLEM/ WHO IS THE CLIENT

"I just haven't been feeling myself lately."

"The teacher says my son is acting up in class, and he has been giving me a hard time at home. I wonder if you could talk to him and straighten him out."

"The judge ordered me to come here for counseling until you say I don't have to. I don't think I need to; it's my ex-wife who's the one with the problems."

"My husband and I agree that our daughter has a problem with her attitude, but personally, I think the real problem is that my husband is never home."

People come to you because of problems and, as brief, solution-focused approaches and managed care have emphasized, it's vital that you know exactly what the problems are. This means having a clear understanding of just what the client is talking about and struggling with: What does "not feeling myself," "acting up in class," or "a problem with attitude" mean? At face value, these are not solvable problems because the behaviors, emotions, and symptoms they indicate are vague, undefined. By helping clients become clearer and more precise about what they are saying, you help them become clearer and more precise about what they are thinking and feeling. This not only begins to bring the problem into the room and to create a clearer picture of what is wrong, but it also helps you begin formulating a clear, positive vision of what can be.

You also need to be clear about who has the problem. Sometimes, especially when the client is a self-referred adult, the client in the room and the client with the problem are one and the same, and it's all pretty simple: "I feel depressed; I'm here so you can help me"; "My kids are running all over me; I need to learn how to handle them better." Other times, however, it's not quite so easy. Often the only person with the problem is the person who is seeing a problem in someone else: the mother who thinks her son should find new friends, but the son thinks his friends are just fine; the father who thinks the mother should be tougher, but the mother feels she has a close relationship with her daughter and the father is just jealous; the wife who wants her husband to stop drinking so much, but he says that he only has a beer now and then and it isn't a problem for anyone but her. If only this other person would change, each says, I would feel better.

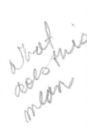

When they all show up in your office, with everyone pointing the finger at someone else, it's important to pair problems and people carefully. The mother and teacher who are having problems with the boy may be the only ones having problems; that is, the boy and father may not be. The man referred by court doesn't have a problem except perhaps with the court order itself; so far the only person with a problem is the judge or probation officer. The father has a problem with his daughter, but the mother has more of a problem with the father. Whoever sees or feels the problem owns it and is ultimately responsible for solving it.[1]

---

[1]Another useful way of approaching varying presentations and levels of motivation is to keep in mind Steve de Shazer's notion of visitor, complainant, and customer. See his *Patterns of Brief Therapy: An Ecosystemic Approach*, Guilford Press, 1982.

When the problem behaviors seem so obvious—the husband is falling down drunk every night; the little boy is fighting everyone in the neighborhood; the teenager is refusing to go to school—it's easy for you to get caught up in everyone's concern and to join forces with them in trying to convince, the identified patient (I.P.), that a problem really does exist. It's an awkward role that you need to avoid. You're stepping out of the service role, rapidly becoming an enforcer, and the I.P. generally starts to respond to you with more and more resistance. From his or her point of view, he or she simply doesn't have a problem, at least not the problem that everyone is so concerned about, and your siding with the others only makes you more quickly dismissed.

Rather than wrestling with the I.P. over the problem, you can have those with the problem come in with the I.P. and talk with different words and a different emotional tone (thanks to you) about their worry and fears about the I.P.'s behavior and see if helps motivate the I.P. to look at the problem. If the person defining the problem—the probation officer, the social service worker, the teacher, or generally some other representative of an agency or institution—isn't present at that first meeting, invite him or her come in. I'm concerned, says the teacher, that if you don't settle down in class and pay attention, you'll be left back. I'm worried, says the mother, that if you don't stop arguing with me at home that you won't behave well with your aunt and shouldn't go to see her this summer. If you don't get counseling to help you control your anger, says the probation officer, not only will you be possibly sentenced to jail time, but you could lose custody of your daughter.

Your other option is to leave the I.P. alone and help the other person see what he or she can do about his or her problem. Thank the son for coming in, set up a time to meet with the mother alone to talk about parenting, and have her sign a release for you to talk to the teacher so that they can coordinate how they will handle the boy's behavior. Tell the client that you'd be happy to tell the court that he doesn't see a need for coming and that they need to consider some other option. Tell the man that you're not sure whether he has a drinking problem or not, but suggest to the wife that she attend an Al-Anon meeting or offer to help her figure out what she can do if the drinking continues.

Your job in this type of confrontation, again, isn't to take sides, but to clarify just what the sides are. The boy, it turns out, is actually very upset that his mother seems to be spending all her time with the new baby, or he feels like his teacher is always on his back and never gives him credit for what he does well. The man agrees that maybe he does have a problem with his temper, but he's gotten a lot worse since he lost his job, and he feels like no one is willing to help him get into job training.

There are now two, or more, problems—the parents' problem and the kid's problem, the agency's problem and the client's problem, the husband's problem and the wife's problem—to work on. That's normal in family therapy simply because there are many people, each with his or her own version of reality. In order to manage them all you start by drawing lines of responsibility around each one, and then do one of several things. You may decide to handle each one separately: "This session we will talk about ways of using time-outs with Billy, and next week maybe we can talk about that holiday depression that you're worried about"; "Let's work on deciding what to do about Mary's school behavior, and then we can work on some of those marital issues."

You can also move to a different level, harness the family's energy, and use systems theory to show the family how two or more problems are connected: "Susan, you don't like Jesse going out with the guys so much, and Jesse, you feel that Susan's always involved with the kids and doesn't want to spend time with you alone. Maybe one problem dovetails into the other"; "John, you're worried about Billy setting fires, and Billy, you're mad at your dad for ignoring you; I wonder if the fires are a way to let your dad know that you're mad and get him to pay attention"; "Manuel, you are worried about Teresa's school work. Teresa, you are upset about your parents arguing so much. I'm thinking that the tension at home may be making you feel depressed and stressed, Teresa, and making it hard to do your work."

This way of connecting of one problem to another is thinking even more like a family therapist and beginning to map the family's patterns. It helps the family members begin to see how their behaviors are interrelated, how one problem is actually an attempted solution to another. By describing the connection, the issue changes, the focus shifts from arguing over who has the problem to finding ways of breaking the pattern. It also builds on the motivation already present as the change in one member's highest concern is indelibly linked to the concerns of the other.

Finally, rather than taking turns working on separate problems and linking problems, it is often possible to collapse several problems into one new one. Jamal, for example, is referred by the school for truancy and comes to the first session with his parents. It is quickly revealed that the father has started gambling heavily again after years of restraint, and the mother reports that she has been suffering with chronic back pain for the past six months, which doctors have done little to help. While on the surface you can look at these as separate problems, it is no coincidence perhaps that they have all erupted since the sudden death of Jamal's six-year-old sister to leukemia last year. In this light it's useful to see their problems are different (albeit not necessarily adaptive) ways of coping with the grief that they all share. By exploring, saying this, and making their loss the focus of the family, the family members are able, with your support, to face their underlying sadness directly and together, rather than getting lost in the specifics of their behaviors. The emotional knot of grief that both links them and handicaps them can begin to unravel.

Similarly, Ann is referred for breaking probation and staying out on the street. The mother also complains that 12-year-old Carl is fighting all the time with his younger brother Sam. All these separate problems are linked, you believe, to the parents' struggle to create structure and consistent limits within the home, and this, in turn, stems from the parents' differing views on the way the children should be handled at all. Again the separate problems are boiled down to a different primary one, namely, the couple's relationship and difficulty working together. This becomes the focus of the therapeutic contract.

Giving the family a new problem to replace the old, worn-out ones that they are stuck on psychologically frees and stimulates new energy and creativity for solving it. The only tricky part for you as the therapist is making sure that the family members agree with the connection you are making between this new problem and their old one. Everyone needs to agree that there really is a link among the grief and Jamal's truancy, Dad's depression, and Mom's back pain, or among the marital strain, Ann's behavior, and the boy's fighting. You can do this through psychoeducation, by exploring and showing the problem in the room (e.g., pointing out how the parents are disagreeing right there and how the kids are acting up or not listening), by the weight of your own expertise, and by their desire to hear your opinion. But sometimes this notion that seemingly disconnected problems are in fact linked can be a hard sell, and you may have to work on the problems separately until you can gather more evidence to convince them that the connection really exists.

Developing a therapeutic contract often starts with negotiation over the problem; before you start negotiating be clear about who the client is and what the problem is.

2. LOOK FOR WHAT'S MISSING

There is a Sherlock Holmes story about a horse that's stolen from a barn one night. Holmes declares to Watson that key to the case is the barking dog. But, says Watson, there was no barking dog. Precisely! says Holmes. The fact that the dog didn't bark meant that whoever came that night was not a stranger, but someone who the dog knew well.

You too need to think like Holmes. You need to see not only what the family presents, but what they don't: to look for what's not being said, what's not happening, what's missing in the picture the family creates of themselves in front of you. These are the holes in the fabric of the family—the father who doesn't come to the appointment, the good things that Michael can do, talking about the time the mother was in jail, the affair the wife had three years ago, anger, sadness, the oldest brother's ongoing depression, laughter, literal pats on the back and physical affection—all the things different members of the family can't do, avoid, aren't aware of.

Or what they can't quite say. This is the subtle awareness of language: the way the father mentions "problems" or "things in the past," how the mother stops and shifts gears in midsentence—"And then he . . . but the teacher said"—or simply trails off. To be aware of this is to see language working as protection. To talk about "a problem" rather than specifically describing the behavior or situation is to put a protective glaze over the emotions. To stop in midsentence and shift course is literally to "not go there." So go there! Ask "What problems?" "What things?" Ask the client to go back and finish the sentence. The more specific the language becomes, the more defined become the emotions.

This seeing what's not there in the room—the people, the emotions, behaviors, the topics, the language—is a way of dropping a line into the deeper emotional waters of the family and discovering what is submerged. You're able to see and guide the family toward where they need to go—the blind spots, the uncharted territory where both their anxiety and healing lie. Since often the most important conversations are the ones that the family avoids, try having them and see what happens: "Tom, you're always so quiet, and I bet Ann thinks you just don't care. Can you tell Ann what you're thinking about what she said?" "It seems you all have never talked about your father's death. Maybe we can all talk about it even for a few minutes." "Helen, you are always in charge of putting Thomas in bed. How about you let John be in charge of doing it this week." "Angie, you made a comment about your jail time. Can you tell me more about that?" By moving toward these areas, you are helping the family members move against their own grain, out of their comfort zones of their patterns. As they approach their anxiety, they can experience change.

And when you feel overwhelmed or unfocused in a session, look for what's missing right there in the room (what is not being talked about, what emotions are being avoided, what secret is lying somewhere in the corner of the family's past) or focus once again on the holes already mapped out (the mother's anger, the father's sadness, the child's inability to say what he or she feels). You are the change-agent and guide. Step forward so the family can do the same.

How do you learn to see and hear what is missing, rather than only what is present? By training your eye, ear, and mind. As you listen to an audiotape, listen for the opposite, for what is not mentioned, for what is only vaguely said. As you watch a videotape, notice what the individuals and the family as a whole are not doing. Like Sherlock Holmes, ask yourself what you would expect to see or hear that you're not. With practice what's presented will become an automatic springboard for zeroing in on what's not there.

3. BLOCK THE DYSFUNCTIONAL PATTERNS

As mentioned earlier, patterns are the heart of family therapy, the way of organizing what you see, the complement to what you don't. The missing elements of family interactions—unexpressed emotions, undiscussed secrets, and so forth—point to anxiety that is too great for the family to handle. On the other hand, dysfunctional behaviors or routines signal that the family has found a way to contain the anxiety provoked by underlying problems. If in what's missing is where the family's anxiety is found, it's in the patterns that the family's anxiety is contained.

The fact that the patterns are contained in what the family presents doesn't necessarily mean they're easy to see. The family doesn't usually think and talk in terms of patterns; they talk in terms of separate, isolated behaviors and events—Eric fights all the time, my husband is always yelling at me. If they do link events, they're usually individual, sequential ones (Johnny starts to complain, then he wails, then he starts kicking, then he falls down on the floor) rather than the horizontal, interactional, bouncing-off-each-other ones that you are looking for. It's your job to find these.

There are two basic ways of doing this. One is to ask "What happens next" questions that help the client map the patterns for you: "So after Johnny starts to complain, what do you generally do? And then he wails, and what do you do then?" By doing this both you and the client are able to see the ping-pong of moves, the connection between the behavior of one and the behavior of the other. Generally the pattern runs until there is a shift in emotion (the mother swats Johnny and he starts to cry, or the mother stomps into her bedroom and slams the door) setting off a new pattern of reconciliation.

The other way of detecting patterns is to see them in the room in the process. Mom tells Susan to sit up straight, Susan slumps even more, Dad tells Susan to listen to her mother, Susan snaps at her father, Mom shrugs and looks away, Susan sits up a bit, slumps again, and it's over. This may be repeated with different content: Mom asking Susan to tell what happened yesterday, Susan saying there's nothing to tell, Dad scolding Susan, and so on. If the pattern isn't automatically reenacted there in the room, ask them to enact for you what happens at home: Ask Dad and daughter to discuss right now a curfew time, ask Mom and son to negotiate a chore list—and watch what enfolds. As it does, you can begin to point out the pattern that you see, in a calm, nonaccusatory way: "It's interesting. I notice that when Susan does _____, you, Mom, always do _____, and then, Dad, you seem to _____." You're introducing the family to ways their reactions have become set.

Once you figure out what the pattern is, your next step is easy: *Block the pattern.* Many newcomers to family therapy go into a panic because they worry that they need to have a healthy pattern already on deck to replace the dysfunctional one. You can do so, of course, and noticing what's missing will give you a direction. But even if you can't think on your feet, by blocking the pattern you will force the family to do something different. So ask Dad not to back up mom and let her and Susan work it out.

Hold up your hands like a traffic cop when the parents begin to double-team their 14-year-old with criticism yet again, and see what happens. While their first reaction is likely to be to ignore you, or to slide back into the safe zone within two seconds, if you persist, continuing to cut them off at the pass, the anxiety of the moment will push them to try a new and different way of relating. This places them in the position of creating their own change, and allows you once again to simply fine-tune it.

4. TRACK THE PROCESS

Content and process: the water versus the flow of water, what the sentence says and the fact that the sentence is a sentence, the complaints about the weekend and the act of complaining—two sides of the whole of what happens in the room. The clinician, like a movie director, pans in and out, back and forth between content (What did the doctor say? What is Dad's specific worry about Karen's dating? What is the family's history of depression?) and the process (the fact that Dad is dominating the conversation, that Mom always sounds hesitant, that the family changes the subject when you bring up the grandfather, or that Andy is sitting silently in the corner).

Different clinical theories place different emphases upon content. Cognitive theory, for example, starts with content and always returns to it: John may feel rejected, but he can learn to tell himself that it doesn't mean that he is a *bad* person or did anything *horrible*. Tim's failing summer school is a *problem*, not a *disaster*. Mike doesn't *always* blow up, but only when he feels that people are understanding how important his career is to him. We may not be able to choose our emotions, but, say cognitive-behavioral therapists, we can choose our thoughts, and the medium of thoughts is language. It's the language of our self-talk that locks, binds, and limits; its distortions create a distorted reality and negative emotions. By remaining alert to this dysfunctional language and consciously changing it, we can directly shape our emotions and change our actions.[2]

Content is also the starting point of therapy—describe the problem, tell me what past treatment you received, let me read the psychological

---

[2]The classic text on cognitive-behavioral theory is Aaron Beck, *Cognitive Therapy and the Emotional Disorders*, Plume, 1979.

report. Content is how the client talks and thinks about problems; it's the currency that builds rapport; it enables us to put together the pieces of the puzzle as the client and others see it. Later on, when therapy is underway, what you, the clinician, say and choose to talk about comes to shape what the client thinks about. Your words come inside, or, to paraphrase Milton Erickson, your voice goes with the client.

But content also rides upon the process. Process is content in motion; process is the raw material of patterns; patterns represent process cut into anxiety-binding shapes. Like a verbal Geiger counter, words tick away with intensity as the client moves toward anxiety. When the words spoken are new words, they have the power to plow open new emotional ground or slowly hack their way through to some new "Aha" insight; they have the power to change the emotional climate in the room. Content is most valuable, most potent, most heard, when it can change this climate, can merge with the process itself: "I'm hesitating and fumbling because I'm afraid that if I say the wrong thing you're going to get mad"; "I hear what you are saying but don't really understand what you're saying; tell me again with different words why my going out last weekend hurt your feelings." This matching of content and process in the moment is the basis of Carl Rogers's concept of authenticity; of Zen consciousness, of self-awareness, -reflection, and -esteem; the key to absolute honesty and living in the present. Powerful stuff.

Like a lot of things, all that power suggests that it is not necessarily easy to attain. In everyday life this merging of content and process rarely happens. Instead content and process exist in separate worlds. The content's ticking slows and eventually slacks off into silence. The words lose their vitality, and become sluggish, overweight verbiage whose only purpose is to sit on anxiety and flatten it, or fill up as much space as possible to keep the anxiety away. Rather than saying that you feel awkward or frightened and don't really know what to say—what is going on with you right there in the room—you punt and talk about the weather, the ball game. You say what you think they want to hear and your emotions are never really acknowledged at all. Even though the words can form a message, the real message that lies in the process, in the moment, is ignored.

This is one of therapy's and therapists' mandates: to go where others fear to tread. A good therapist is always turning up the corners of the content to peek underneath and catch the mismatch of word and intent, to separate medium from the message. Your ability to realize what's happening while it's happening—the father is distracting, the daughter is looking hurt but sounding angry, the mother is trying to pull rank by bringing up the past—should be one of your strengths. This is a skill that your training and sensitivity have prepared you to do and your courage allows you to accomplish.

When the content seems overwhelming or without meaning, it is the process, like the patterns and holes and problems, that you can return to and center upon. It enables you to step back and take the long shot, see and change the patterns as they are unfolding, "catch" yourself and pull yourself out of the swirl, and consciously put on the brakes. Even though most of us, including the families we see, are good at recognizing the process in others—"There he goes again, always interrupting me"—the skill becomes lost in seeing it in ourselves or in relationships where the patterns and process are so powerful. Your view as an outsider is invaluable.

By focusing on the process in the room, the family becomes aware again that there *is* a process. By your example they learn to separate process from content, see that the water and the flow of the water are different yet intimately connected, that the changing of one will change the other. Shifting the focus to the process helps the family not only to see the patterns as they are played out right before them, but also to experience what it is like to step back and out of them at the same time. Once this shift in focus is demonstrated and experienced, the family members can begin to learn to do the same on their own.

As with calling attention to patterns, it's your job as the therapist to take the risk, and it is a risk, to shift the focus to the process when content no longer represents what's occurring. This is usually done with questions ("John, you're talking about the good times of the past, but looking mighty sad. How are you feeling right here, right now?") or statements ("Mary, I'm trying right now to offer a suggestion and I feel like you're ignoring me"). The client, be it one individual or the entire family, has to shift, and is forced to stop and think about what just happened and is happening right then. This shift in focus creates the opportunity for the family members to move from meaningless content to meaningful, honest content that fully incorporates the underlying emotions.

Often, however, as with initial stopping of patterns, the client's first reaction to your intervention is to resist you in order to reduce his or her anxiety? "I *was* listening" Mary mumbles back, both denying the reality in the present and avoiding the confrontation. But if you stick with the process? ("Did you just feel like I was scolding you?" said in a gentle voice) and help the client to stay focused on what's happening in the present, cut him or her off from slipping back into the same content, the client not only plows new emotional ground within the relationship with you, but he or she begins both to discriminate content from process and to learn to move between them.

Tracking the process allows you to keep a handle on what's always going on simply by asking and focusing on it. You can immediately see the impact and effectiveness of your interventions—the story changes or stops, the anger shifts to sadness—and you can gauge the pacing. By tracking the process both you and the client can learn to tackle problems and derailments—the hurt feelings, the misunderstood comment, which are sources of resentment in the therapeutic and family relationships— right there and then, directly and immediately as they unfold. The therapy stays on course, and the family sees how to confront problems quickly and effectively. By staying aware of and on the growth edge, you and the client can avoid creating and lapsing into your own stale patterns of behavior that can bind anxiety and blunt the change making.

Finally, process is ultimately what therapy is. Often new therapists feel overwhelmed because they believe that they need to reshape the client's larger world, a feeling that usually parallels the client's sense that everything is "out there" and falling on his or her head. But the "out there" can only be managed in the right here, right now. Your influence and power is limited to what you do and say and can create there in the room within the micro-process of interactions between you. All of the client's world and problems are encapsulated there in the patterns and interactions right before you. This is all you can work with and have available to work with; this is where your skills are concentrated and applied. Everything else—whether the client follows your advice, pays the rent, or controls his temper with the kids at home—is out of your immediate control. Your challenge is shape the time, space, and interactions in the immediacy of the moment to create something new.

This is often a difficult perspective to absorb and, at times, to maintain. When we are feeling frustrated or overwhelmed we need to remind ourselves both of the limits of our power and that the concentration of our power is there in the present and in the room. By doing this, we teach families to do the same: To think and act now, rather than waiting for the future; to move against the grain of their hesitations, avoidance, self-doubt, and/or self-criticism and speak clearly what is in their hearts; to realize that the work of good relationships over the long term is more about having healthy ways of tackling problems and changes and less about the content or outcome of any specific one; that life happens in the present and can be measured in the quality of our interactions. These are among the most powerful and basic of life's lessons.

5. EXPERIENCE BEFORE EXPLANATION

The focus on process, patterns, and what's missing tells us that you can see before you both the creation of the problem and its possible solution. The focus on who and what the problem is tells us that the more you can link what you do in the room with what goes on in the family's life outside the room, the more therapy is seen by the family as a viable and active means of changing the problem, rather than becoming merely more talk about it. What ties these two foci together is the clinician's skillful use of that set of twins, experience and explanation. *Experience*, the close cousin of process, is the one who runs through the room intent on what happens; *explanation*, the close cousin of content, is the one who smoothes and soothes, who makes sense out of what experience has just done, and connects it to the family's problem and needs.

Just as the clinician learns to move between content and process, he or she moves between these two twins. A good balance is important. Let experience run too wild, too long, and the family feels overwhelmed, shaky, fragmented, frightened; everything is in shambles, their anxiety goes through the roof, and more often than not they run away and don't come back. Too much explanation and the family goes to sleep; like its cousin, content, on a bad day explanation bores the family to death; the words wash over them, leaving them unchanged.

Explanation's strength is its calming presence, immensely valuable when lowering anxiety is exactly what you want. This is what the doctor does when she tells the frightened little boy that she is going to give him a shot in his arm and it's going to sting for a minute, or describes to the obsessing patient exactly what will happen in surgery tomorrow, and what it will be like after surgery while he's there in the hospital. This what you do in the first session when you talk to the family about what therapy can or cannot do regarding the problem, or what the format will be for the session.

The psychodynamic approaches devoted a great amount of attention to beefing up explanation's power and ability to mobilize change. These explanations were renamed in their vocabulary "interpretations," and like the puny David facing Goliath, their lack of experience's kinetic power is made up for with impeccable timing. Properly timed interpretations are, in the psychodynamic process, an art form. When hurled at just the right moment these explanations strike the client right between the eyes, crystallizing all that the client has been moving toward in awareness. They shine a light on the vague shadows that the client has been slowly groping through; suddenly, the shadows dissolve into something clear and hard. The client has more than an explanation; he or she has an "insight," an "Aha" experience that then can spill over into emotions and behaviors. Good interpretations transform explanations into experience.

The down side to this process is the length of time it takes. The less directive role of the psychodynamic therapist means that he or she is essentially waiting for Goliath to approach, waiting for the unconscious process to built and take hold. The directive role of the family therapist speeds up this process; rather than waiting, he or she marches forward into the fray and begins to stop the patterns, pushes the family to see what's missing. These actions raise anxiety and open up the possibility of change.

All this leads us to the fifth basic concept: Experience before explanation. If the primary goal is to get the family moving, to ride on the motivation that brought them into the office, they need, to paraphrase Fritz Perls, the founder of Gestalt therapy, an experience, not an explanation. Bring the problem alive, get them to try something different, talk about what they don't want to talk about, have them taste something new— then mop up with explanation. What you're then doing is exactly what the psychodynamic therapist has been waiting to do for months, providing an explanation that crystallizes and shapes the anxiety that you have just generated. If explanation walks into the room with a bucket and mop too soon, while everything is still orderly and set, he stands in the corner and melts into the woodwork. Everyone wonders why he's there.

By marching ahead with experience you're not only breaking up the patterns, but desensitizing the family to the experience of change, to the taking of risk. Rather than yet-again retreating from new situations, or, out of fear, seeing the new as only another example of the old, the family approaches their anxiety with your help; when they do so they increase both their self-esteem and courage.

Of course, you, as the clinician, are once again the best person to model this courage. Armed with your theory and philosophy, you are the one best able to push into the holes that you see the family cautiously walking around, that you sense by feeling the edges of your own anxiety. While this may sound daunting, it needn't be. Here are some examples of experience before explanation:

This mother is angry. For the last six months her 11-year-old son has been driving her crazy—getting into fights at school, earning failing grades, arguing with her all the time. She thinks the problem is the new kid in his class that he has been hanging around with. Had anything happened six months ago? you ask. No, she says, then hesitates. Well, she says matter-of-factly, his grandmother, my mother, died back during the summer, but she had been ill for a long time, and we all knew it was coming. Tell me about your mother, you say. She begins to describe her, and as she does her eyes become teary. Do you miss her? you ask quietly. The wall around her grief begins to break, and she quietly begins to sob for many minutes; you sit with her and wait. When she finally calms down and looks at you again, you ask, Do you think your son feels the same way you do? I don't know, I guess, but we never talk about it, she responds. I wonder, you say, if the way he has been acting is connected to all this sadness and the way you both have been feeling.

At the urging of the school teacher, Jim brings in his eight-year-old daughter, Jenny, who has lately become moody and withdrawn. He is not so much concerned about why, but what he should do about it. The parents have been divorced for several years, but, Jim assures you, they continue to have a good relationship, and Jenny has handled it well. Jim has been steadily and recently dating a woman named Cathy. He swears that Jenny likes Cathy, though Jenny says little to anyone, including you. You ask her to draw a picture of her family, and with some prodding she does. You show it to the father. There, clearly labeled in her eight-year-old scrawl, is a picture of her mother and father holding hands with a smiling Jenny standing right in the middle of them.

It's the classic marital argument. Lisa starts complaining how Phil is always criticizing her, and Phil snaps back, saying that she never follows through on what she agrees to do. Quickly they escalate using sarcasm, making faces, yelling, and bringing up old wounds and stories of the past. You hold up your hands and ask them both to stop. You ask Lisa to turn her chair toward you, and ask her to say more about what bothers her when Phil seems to be critizing her. She becomes teary and says she feels pushed away, lonely, much like she did when her father did the same thing when she was growing up. You talk briefly about the power of triggers from the past and ask her to tell Phil how she would like him to speak to her when he is frustrated.

Again we see the other basic concepts coming into play: clarifying the problem, focusing on process, moving toward what's missing, breaking patterns. But what each example also shows is the creating of experience in order to set the stage for explanation. You may have guessed the moment that the mother mentioned the death of her mother that the grief may be trickling beneath the boy's acting out. You could have cut to the chase and explained this to the mother, who most likely would have nodded her head, but emotionally disagreed and discounted what you were saying simply because of the anxiety it created.

But by gently leading the mother into her grief, the telling of the story of her son and her mother flow together. Only after she is emotionally aware of her grief can she consider it resting within her son as well; only then does your linking them together and redefining the problem in new terms now make sense and seem relevant to her.

The same is true with the father and daughter. The father wanted to know what to do, and you could have quickly given him a list of behavioral things to try at home. What's missing, however, is the content of the daughter's silence, his own reluctance to look underneath the changes in his family, or the impact of his new relationship. The daughter's picture powerfully and directly says to him what your explanation would not.

Finally, it's easy to see how the couple's verbal and nonverbal behavior is fueling old patterns of destruction. Rather than giving a mini-lecture on their poor communication (and possibly replicating the criticizing process). you break the patterns and give Lisa a chance to talk and Phil to listen, without all the nonverbal and verbal triggers. More importantly, you help them create a different, positive interaction right there in the room that you can then map out for them so that they can replicate it at home. Should it not work—should Phil fail to listen or dismiss what Lisa says—you can see where and how it breaks down, and try something else.

What each of these examples have in common is the shift in the emotional climate in the room. It is said that one can't solve a problem with the same emotion that fostered it or with the same consciousness that created it. Only by changing the emotional climate in the room is the family able to see what you see and fully absorb the new ideas you have to offer, which in turn can help them change their perceptions of the problem.

If you are moving too quickly and notice that the client's anxiety is rising too high and creating resistance (e.g., not paying attention, distracting, outright refusing to try what you suggest), you can use explanation as a brake: "Lisa, I'm asking you to look at me rather than Phil so that you can say what you think without getting distracted by his nonverbal behavior"; "Jim, I asked Jenny to draw a picture because it is usually easier for kids to say how they feel through art or play"; "Mrs. Johnson, I'm asking about your mother because I'm wondering how much the loss of his grandmother may be bothering your son even though he doesn't talk about it. Often children's sadness comes out as behavior problems." Statements like these put a frame around the experience and make it just enough less threatening that you can continue to go forward.

There's always the temptation, especially when you feel overwhelmed or frustrated, to use explanations like a blanket to smother the fires of anxiety (yours and the family's) before it gets out of control. But the better way to look at anxiety is to see it as a tightrope that you and the family walk across together. Explanations are the balancing pole that you hold in your hands and gently shift from side to side in order to stay upright and moving along the line. With practice your skill in using the balancing pole increases, and explanations become more and more part of the experience itself.

6. BE PROACTIVE

Good novelists and filmmakers talk about creating the fictive dream, where the reader or moviegoer is drawn into the character's world and emotionally enters the story. The writer's or director's skill and challenge comes in providing the right amounts and quality of description, dialogue, action, and focus to sustain this dream state. When the writer or director fails to do this, the audience becomes conscious of the writing, acting, or camera work, bored, and too aware that they are in fact, reading a book or watching a movie.

As the therapist your challenge is essentially the same—to pull the family into the therapy process and experience, to focus on the patterns and what's missing in a way that keeps them engaged—like a good writer would—rather than bored (which makes them put down the therapy) or too threatened (which makes them slam it shut and run away). You start with the bringing together of "visions," the family's, in the form of expectations and their perception of the problem, and yours, gathered from your unique impressions. The therapy begins with the melding of both visions into one.

As I've been saying all along, this requires that you take the lead, that you be the author, that you take a proactive rather than reactive stance. Families expect this; they look to you for direction, answers, advice. If they see you as acting passively, doubts may be raised about your competence, commitment, or strength to take them on. More importantly, unlike individual work, where the simple presence of the therapist is enough to raise anxiety and push the client out of old patterns, the greater number of people in the family can turn therapist passivity into therapist nonpresence. Without your active interaction, the family quickly falls into its well-worn dysfunctional patterns and recreates the same experience they have at home. They walk out thinking that they could have done the same thing at home for free, and decide that therapy is a waste of time and money.

Being proactive means sharing your vision as soon as possible by setting goals for each session, then stepping back and looking at the process to avoid getting lost in content the way the family does. It doesn't mean being foolhardy, irresponsible, or dangerous, but it does mean being brave enough to try something different, being flexible and pragmatic enough to stimulate change, rather than retreating from change by being too rigid and purist. When you feel stuck, try something else, even if it is to talk about being stuck. Rather than absorbing their helplessness, show the family through your behavior the value and workings of commitment and perseverance in the face of problems. Keep trying and keep moving within the session.

7. BE HONEST

If being proactive keeps you moving, honesty keeps you moving in the right direction. Honesty is the essential ingredient of leadership and your default position. When you fear that things have drifted off course, when you are not sure what is going on or what you are going to do, when you feel confused and worry that (gulp!) you made a mistake, being open and saying this to the family keeps you responsible, models authenticity, reduces the pressure to do it right or have all the answers. You're are not giving up your leadership, you're merely telling the family that it's time to regroup and check the map.

For those new to family therapy, this can seem like a difficult stance to take. It's all too easy to feel that you have to have all the answers, that the family will see you as incompetent, that if you say what you think, they'll get angry, they'll get even more depressed, they won't be able to handle it. But remember that the beauty of family therapy is that you don't have to work so hard, you don't have to be the one to crack the case, to get something absolutely right. By changing the process and patterns you are solving the problem. If you have a question and don't have the answer, don't panic, you're not alone. Throw it back to the family and ask them to figure it out with you. If you feel stuck, ask if they feel the same, see if anyone has any ideas. Family therapy has the potential to become good group therapy; your job is to guide the process and keep everyone on task.

We're back to values, principles, and assumptions. My principles tell me that it is better to show integrity, to match my words and actions and emotions; that my honesty encourages others to be honest as well; that supporting greater integrity and honesty is, when you think about it, what therapy really is all about.

There you have it, the seven basics of family therapy, the core skills that can keep you on track and sane. Match them not only against your own conception of family therapy, but against your own personality and values. In the next three chapters we explore how these basics are applied to the beginning, middle, and end stages of family therapy.

Looking Within: Chapter 4 Exercises

1. It easier to develop skills when you're not under performance pressure. Increase your sensitivity to what's missing, the patterns, and process by watching it in others outside the clinical sessions. Sit back and watch what emerges over the next couple of staff meetings. Look at the nonverbal behavior among people

at the tables around you in a restaurant. See how quickly you can begin to hear and see the holes, how quickly you can tell when a pattern is being repeated, or what the verbal or nonverbal triggers are that set it off.

2. Another exercise in courage building: Try being honest outside the clinical room. Not big honesty in the form of confession, but small honesty in the form of staying attuned to your own inner process as you interact with someone, matching your words and inner feelings. Undoubtedly you do this well already with certain people in your life (your daughter, your spouse, your best friend); try doing it with someone where it is less comfortable (a stranger, your supervisor, one of your parents). Be sure to pat yourself on the back for the effort regardless of how you think it turns out.

3. In a similar vein, practice increasing your awareness of the micro-process between you and another. Practice your listening skills, focusing less on content and more on their process. When he trails off in a sentence, ask him to pick it up again and finish it. When she uses some abstract word, ask her to give you an example to make it more precise and concrete, and see what happens emotionally. Comment on nonverbal behaviors or underlying emotions. Watch the connection and disconnections between you. When you make a statement, see how well he agrees or follows along, or glazes over or dismisses verbally or nonverbally what you had just said. If there is disconnection, stop and fix the problem right there in the room—"It seems like you don't agree," or "You're getting quiet. Are you bored, am I talking too much?" Again, the content is not important; focus instead on the process.

[5]

In the Beginning

GREAT EXPECTATIONS

Meeting someone new is always so awkward. It's easy for you to worry about what may happen: "Will the family start arguing?" "Will they expect me to tell them how to fix their child's encopresis in the first session?" "What if the teenager refuses to talk or stomps out?" On top of that you're already feeling a bit frazzled because your car decided to break down in the middle of the interstate, and then the director has just come around *again*, not too subtly reminding everyone how billing income is down and that, by the way, your performance evaluation is coming up next month. Ugh.

But from the family's side of the room, they've got anxieties of their own: "Will I be liked?"; "Will the kids misbehave and embarrass us?"; "Will I have to talk about my abortion?"; "Is Meg going to bring up that one time I got drunk and slapped her?"; "Is this guy going to think that this is all my fault?"

Yes, beginnings are always difficult for everyone, and the beginnings of therapy are no different. Even the most seasoned clinicians feel a flutter of anxiety when a new family first walks into the office, and it's important that you get off on the right foot—create good impressions, clarify and meet expectations, maintain family motivation, develop and begin an effective treatment plan. This stage is the foundation upon which all that follows is built. It's a time for forming hypotheses, but even more a time of fostering hope. By the time those butterflies have subsided on both sides of the room, both you and the family need to begin to share a vision of what can be, and experience the feeling that this therapy might actually work.

DEADENDS, DETOURS, AND OTHER DANGERS

Allen and Terry Adamson come in with their two sons, Daniel, age 12, and Brian, 10. The boys are constantly at each other's throats, says Dad, and to cap it all off Daniel was recently caught breaking into a neighbor's house with a couple of his friends. Both parents agree that the boys haven't gotten along since Brian was old enough to crawl, but things have been especially difficult the last six months. They had tried therapy one time before, a few months back, but only went once. All the therapist did was ask a bunch of questions, gave no suggestions, and only seemed interested in scheduling another appointment. They thought it was a waste of time.

Here you have your presenting problem. Your mind is probably already racing ahead, formulating, based upon your theory, possible hypotheses and questions to ask. But before you begin worrying about all the things you need to do, it's helpful stop for a minute and think about what would be important for you *not* to do. Here are some suggestions:

• *Don't wait to begin treatment.* We all learn about assessment and treatment, Act 1, Act 2, one logically following from the other. While it's good to think this way, in the real world of managed care and brief therapy, assessments are usually one-session affairs with treatment beginning by the time the family walks out of the room, if not earlier.

Most families expect this from you as well. I once worked at an agency where a questionnaire was handed out to all new clients at their first appointment asking them about their expectations of counseling. When asked how many times they thought they would need to come, most (over 60%) thought they would need to come two, three times; a sizable minority (over 30%) thought they would need to come only once. These clients imagined sitting down, telling the therapist their problem, the therapist giving them a diagnosis and some advice, and they're done. Not much different from going to see their family doctor.

With that expectation nothing could be more exasperating for a family than to spend 15 minutes filling out forms, and then another 35 min-

utes answering question after question, some of which seem to them totally unrelated to the problem ("So how do you get along as a couple?";
"Any complications during pregnancy?"), only to have the therapist suddenly look at her watch and say, "Wow, looks like we ran out of time. Let's
continue this next week. How about same time?" and send the family on
their way. As soon as they hit the hallway, they're thinking, "Continue
what? Wasting my time?!" No surprise when they don't show up the next
week.

Before that first session ends, families like the Adamsons are expecting not only to be heard, but also to hear something useful—what you
think is going on, who's really got the problem, what fancy test you're going to do next time to tell what is really going on, what they should do
this week when the fighting breaks out again—something. To walk out
feeling that they just covered the exact same ground that they did with
the other therapist, leaves them wondering what's different this time, why
they bothered to come.

Think of treatment as not coming after assessment as much as running alongside it. Treatment, in fact, becomes part of the assessment process. By making a homework assignment, for example, you not only give
the family a way to work on the problem, but you give yourself a way of
finding out what works (or doesn't work) with this particular family. By
asking the mother to say something positive to her daughter, rather than
constantly criticizing, right there in the room, you are able to see how
willing she is to follow your suggestions, how hard it is for her to actually
do it, and whether switching from nagging to praise actually helps change
the daughter's reactions.

If your assessment does need to take a certain amount of time (e.g.,
you want the psychiatrist to do a neuropsychological evaluation; you want
to do a session of play therapy with the child who wouldn't talk in the session), clearly describe the time frame for the family so that they know
when to expect some feedback. Demonstrate leadership.

• *Don't continue to replicate dysfunctional patterns.* While it's important to get a clear idea of the interactional patterns in the family, either by
description or better yet by observation, it's equally important to stop
them, especially those tied to the presenting problem. If dysfunctional
patterns continue for too long in the session, the family is going to feel
that therapy isn't much different from what they do at home for free.

What does this mean for the Adamsons? If the parents' complaint is that the boys are fighting too much at home, you don't want to allow the boys to argue for too long in the office, nor have the parents repeat over and over again their ineffective way of handling it, such as scolding the boys but not stopping them. Similarly, if a wife complains to you in the session that her husband is always running her life and putting her down, you don't want him to go on too long about how incompetent he thinks she is or how she needs to figure out why she's so sensitive. This only replicates the problem and process that they are already habituated to; your silence, by default, sanctions it and keeps it going.

Silence is never neutral. While you're thinking that you are taking time to observe, or doing your best not to take sides, your silence is subtly reinforcing the process in the room. If that process is destructive (the couple is "fighting dirty" by bringing up the that affair from 20 years ago; the parents suddenly start to pick on the family scapegoat rather than talking about their own problems as a couple; someone is threatening physical harm to another or emotionally getting out of control), your silence, taken as support, will only escalate the destructive process further. Not only does your lack of action make it harder for you to step in eventually interrupt the process, but you will have also damaged your credibility as a leader.

Even before the session begins, think about ways the presenting problem could be enacted within the session. Once you see how the destructive patterns unfold, be prepared to stop them.

• *Don't leave anyone out.* If you only talk to the parents and get their view of the problem, or join the parents in scolding Daniel about the break-in, the boys will write you off as just another adult who's going to act like a cop. Similarly, if you allow Mrs. Adamson to go on and on about anger at her husband or her sadness about her dead father, the others present in the room, even if they are concerned about her or momentarily relieved that they don't have to talk, will also feel left out, ignored, or jealous of the attention you are giving her. You may have to work harder to pull them in later, and the family will leave with a distorted sense of what is the most important focus. Make some contact with everyone in the room, bring them into the process, get their views about the problem.

• *Don't overcontrol the flow of the conversation.* The first few sessions are a balancing act between assessment and treatment, content and process, the most dominant person in the family and the others present—and also between your leading and following. You want to gather the information you need to confirm your hypothesis, stop the dysfunctional patterns, point the family in a new direction. You want to take charge, but not so much that you train the family to be passive. They shouldn't expect that you will always ask the questions, have the answers, run the show.

Rather than seeing yourself as driving the car that is the family, think of yourself as the driving instructor in the passenger seat. In the beginning you have to instruct more—setting down rules, clarifying expectations, showing them what buttons to push, what controls to use. But once everything is underway and rolling, once they gain experience in running the process, you can begin to sit back. Your job is to help the family stay on the road, caution them when they are swerving too far into a power struggle or into the ditch of passivity, encouraging them to look ahead and anticipate the dangers. Occasionally you may be forced to step in and use your own brake to slow things down to avert a collision, but you never grab the steering wheel out of their hands and drive them yourself. Over time the sessions become more and more their own. Your list of questions gets shorter, the sermonettes more rare. Your focus shifts from their fundamental ability to control the car toward more advanced skills of performance driving. You point out the turns that lead them out of their familiar psychological neighborhoods onto less familiar paths toward their anxiety, change, and growth.

In order to get to that point, you want the therapy to move as quickly as possible toward what it will realistically become, give the family in those first few sessions a good taste of what therapy's like beyond the gathering of histories and the filling out of forms. If you are too controlling, bombarding the family with question after question, feeling responsible for coming up with ideas about what to talk about, always initiating, always being the one to have the answers rather than helping the family figure them out for themselves, you'll quickly feel overwhelmed and eventually run out of steam. And the family, not knowing anything else, will never have learned to drive themselves.

What usually propels all this overregulation is your fear—of the family's disapproval, of losing control, of chaos breaking out if you hold the reins too loosely, causing the process to stampede over a cliff. Learning to take a looser grip on the reins begins with a basic trust in the family, and in yourself: a trust that the family will not only learn, but also take responsibility for their lives; trust that therapy is an effective partnership that develops over time; trust that in the worst-case scenario your courage and honesty will in themselves be enough to manage whatever may come up. The next step is in taking the risk, stopping your own pattern of control— holding back on all the questions, letting the family members talk—and discovering what happens to yourself as well as them when you do. Once you find out that your worst fears don't come true—the family doesn't hate you, the marital explosion isn't all that explosive, the stomping-out teenager comes back within a few minutes—you become less afraid, freer to experiment with your power and skills, more confident and flexible in what you do; not surprisingly, the family begins to learn to do the same.

In looking over this list of things to avoid it's easy to see that what you're avoiding is getting off on the wrong foot: the family's, by replicating the problem, by taking sides, or by being too passive, or your own, by taking too much responsibility and control. This is what the beginning stage is all about—getting a good start that creates its own therapeutic momentum. If you can avoid these four dangers, you're halfway there. The other half is knowing what to move toward.

BUILDING RAPPORT

You can ask all the smart questions in the world, but it won't matter if Allen and Terry think that you don't understand or don't care about how they feel or think that you are incompetent. Rapport is the matter of building the relationship, conveying competence and trust, being sensitive to the family's needs and fears as you gently lead them in and out of their anxiety. Without rapport, without an emotional connection to you, your clients will be too frightened and will refuse to move.

So how do you build rapport? You show courtesy, addressing everyone by name, inviting them to sit down, apologizing if you were a few minutes late. You listen to what each person says, give each a chance to speak, and show that you're listening by not interrupting and by making eye contact. You show that you understand not by saying "I understand,," which usually sounds phony, but by inviting them to explain more in order to help you understand: "I'm not quite sure I understand. Can you tell me more . . . ?" You acknowledge the emotions underlying their statements: "Allen, it must be really frustrating for you"; "Terry, you sound really worried about Daniel"; "Daniel, I bet you feel like your folks are always on your back." You can mirror the body posture of the person talking, or use the skills of neurolingusitic programming and talk the language of each person's perceptual system: "Allen, how do you *see* the problem?"; "Terry, how do you *feel* about what Brian just said?"; "Daniel, how do you *handle* it when your dad blows up at you?"

You also build rapport by being sensitive to their racial, ethnic, religious, or cultural differences. In recent years much has been written about culture and its impact on clinical practice. All of us know that the clients' racial, ethnic, religious, and cultural backgrounds shape their expectations of therapy, their family structure and family values, the role of the parents and children, and the ways decisions are made and priorities are set; familiarizing yourself with these cultural differences is an important foundation for your work. But you don't need an encyclopedic knowledge of various cultural values as much as a respectful attitude. This means raising differences rather than dismissing them, showing inquisitiveness and interest in their uniqueness. You can demonstrate this simply by asking questions: "You mentioned that you are Hindu (or Muslim or Jewish or born-again Christian)—can you tell me how your religious beliefs shape your family values?"; "Every family is different—what are some of the values or beliefs that you feel make your family unique and special"; "Because I am not Latino myself, I wonder if you can tell me how your heritage has influenced your family values." Families appreciate the opportunity to discuss their particular view of life. By asking and listening carefully, you are showing respect for their views and a willingness to incorporate them in your working partnership.[1]

Most of all, however, you build rapport by following the basics. You determine who has and what is the problem; Terry's worried about Brian, Allen's mad at Daniel, Daniel is upset about school. You carefully track the process (you ask Allen and Terry to talk in front of you about how to handle Daniel and point out how easily they disagree); you block the dysfunctional patterns once they become apparent (stop the parents from double-teaming Brian when its clear that he only tunes them out more); you educate and explain family process and diagnoses to reduce anxiety and increase awareness ("While we usually think of depression as making people feel sad and slow, sometimes people, especially children, can seem irritable"); you ask questions about what's missing ("You mentioned 'things' in the past—what kind of 'things' are you talking about?"), and

[1] That being said, it can be helpful to have some knowledge of how ethnicity, culture, and race may shape a family's expectations of the therapy process. The classic text for this is Monica McGoldrick et al., *Ethnicity and Family Therapy*, Guilford Press, 2005.

have the courage to move into areas that in everyday conversation others stay away from ("What hurt you most about the divorce?"); you seek to create an experience and change the emotional climate (you point out that Allen looks sad as he talks about his last blowout with the boys and quietly support him as he tears up). You initiate action so they learn that therapy is an active process, more than answering questions and getting advice. You begin to create that vision of what can be by asking them to image it with you. You are as honest as you can be.

Again, it's not having the right answer that's important, but the effort and the willingness to help the family find the right answer. If you can do even some of these things within the first session, the emotional connection, the rapport, will be there.

GATHERING INFORMATION

Throughout the course of family therapy you will be shifting back and forth between (1) time spent in sessions finding out about something you need to know (e.g., Bobby's school history, why the parents got divorced, the grandmother's problems with depression, how well the behavioral chart worked last week), information that helps you better understand the problem and develop or fine-tune a treatment plan, and (2) time spent within the session helping the family reach their goals—providing information about the problem, helping them learn and practice new skills (e.g., the father listening to his son instead of criticizing, the oldest daughter staying out of the fights between the parents), gaining new insights (e.g., helping Mother see how she is treating her oldest daughter more like an adult friend than a teenager), discussing in a safe environment issues important to them (e.g., the big fight over the weekend or couple's sexual problems). Most of what you do will be of the latter type, helping the family reach their goals; most of the information gathering obviously takes place in the beginning stage.

Figuring out what you need to know and finding it out can seem overwhelming. Simply put, there are two types of information you need— about content and about process. Under each of these is the need for generic information, that is, information that you would gather from every family that you see, and specific information, that is, what your theory leads you to explore that would help you confirm your initial hypothesis about the cause of this particular problem with this particular family.

We'll be talking more about specific theories in the second section. For now let's just look at the generic content and process information that you'll need:

Content information

What is the specific presenting problem or problems? Who has the problem? Who in the family or community is most concerned about the problem?

If there is more than one problem, what has the highest priority?

What is the family's theory, theories about the problem?

What has the family tried so far to solve the problem?

What are the family's expectations of therapy? Do the parents see themselves as part of the solution?

What is the larger context and history of the problem? Who else may be involved? What themes seem to constantly reappear?

Process information

How well do the family members communicate with each other (don't talk, have trouble expressing how they feel, interrupt and don't listen, etc.)?

What are the individual family members' reactions to you as the therapist (e.g., intimidated, closed, eager to please, seductive, skeptical, passive, angry, aggressive)?

How anxious are the various family members?

What is the emotional range of the various family members? What emotion is each person most comfortable expressing?

What's missing?

What patterns do you see? What don't you want to replicate?

The reason for listing many of these is obvious (e.g., presenting problem, the family's anxiety); others have been discussed already (e.g., notice what is missing, tracking the patterns). Some, however, are new and require some explanation:

• *Theories about the presenting problem.* One of the first families I ever saw was a poor family living on the father's disability benefits and food stamps. The son, age eight, was having major disciplinary problems at school, and I went to see the family in their home. As I walked through the door into the living room I could see the father in the corner sitting in his wheelchair. He was barking orders to his wife, who looked tired and depressed, but was doing her best to fetch whatever it was her husband wanted. The eight-year-old would periodically slam open the back door, the father would yell at him, the son would ignore him, grab something from the kitchen and slam back out. In the back bedroom was the 11-year-old son, who, it turned out, rarely came out of his room.

I explained to the father why I was there, asked him about the behavioral problems his son was having, and why he thought his son was having so much trouble at school. "You know what his problem is," the father said as he squinted and held his index finger up in the air, "he's allergic to cow's milk. You see when he was a baby he couldn't drink regular cow's milk, and we had to feed him that soy milk. It's that soy milk that messed up his head."

Every family has a theory about the cause of the problem they face, even when they say at first that they have no idea—it's biological or genetic; it's because someone else doesn't like them; it's the result of some past trauma, past karma, God's punishment, poor parenting, something. We all instinctively create some explanation for our problems rather than live with the uncertainty of having none. While it was obvious to me even as a novice that this family had numerous problems for numerous possible reasons, the father's explanation for his son's behavior had already determined for him the solution, namely, that there was none. His son, in his mind, was irreparably damaged (like him, perhaps) by a common childhood event. Given his point of view, this father was not optimistic about my ability to help his son learn to behave, and he saw my questions about his disability and his family as irrelevant and nosy.

Finding out in the first session the family's theory or theories for the problem is important because they tell you where the family believes the solutions lie. Most often the family sees the problem within one person, in this case, within the son. From your perspective as a family therapist your challenge is to expand the definition of the problem to include the involvement of the entire family, to offer new ideas in order to reshape their theory, to experientially connect the problem as they see it to the patterns within the family. Knowing their theory gives you the starting point linking their ideas with your own.

• *What has the family tried to solve the problem?* You are seeking two kinds of information here. The obvious one is finding out what has or hasn't worked (e.g., grounding, ignoring the problem, medication) and eliminating options. Not all problems have to be complex and convoluted. Often the first and best line of approach is plain old problem solving and consulting: Give the family some basic information (e.g., the need for structure and simple directions for a child with attention-deficit/ hyperactity disorder; details about the current treatment approaches to enuresis) and help them decide on the options that they are willing to try. Sometimes what they are already doing (their use of time-outs with Kenisha, the father's combination Alcoholics Anonymous [AA] meetings and increased exercise for his recovery) just needs to be fine-tuned (time-outs need to be shorter or in Kenisha's bedroom; the father needs to increase his meetings when under stress or have daily contact with his sponsor) or to be done more consistently or for a longer period of time so they can take hold.

Other times, with problems involving the children, the actual solution that's described is itself fine, but the parents are not really on the same page; the children wind up splitting the parents or one parent undermines the other. It's helpful not only to ask the parents what solutions they've tried, but how they differ in approach and style: "Which one of you tends to be more firm? Which one of you is more likely to give in if the kids press you hard enough?" These kinds of questions can normalize differences and begin to move the parents toward a more solid joint agreement.

But the other reason for asking about what's been tried is to help you see and understand more about the problem-solving process within this particular family. Not only what is decided, but who decides, who carries out the solution, what happens when someone disagrees, and what causes a reasonable idea to be lost in conversation. Tracking these process questions up front lets you know what problems in the family dynamics get in the way of applying the information and solving the presenting one.

• *Expectations of therapy.* Just as we naturally develop theories about our problems, we all naturally approach new situations with expectations already in mind. I've always been amazed (though I shouldn't be) by the parents who drop their eight- or ten-year-old child off at the front door of the agency for a first appointment. When I ask the child where the parents are, he or she says that they are sitting out in the car listening to the radio, or they needed to go to the grocery store and be out front in an hour, to pick up the child. Similarly, I've met husbands who imagine that you will excuse them after few minutes and have an intimate "girl talk" with their wives to help her to be less nervous about sex, mothers who ask if you can hypnotize their daughters so they will be less obsessed about their boyfriends, or parents who expect that by the end of the first session you'll write a letter to the school principal recommending that their daughter be readmitted back into school.

Some family's expectations are realistic (they will need to come a few times together as a family; you'll help them communicate better) but others (you'll have a talk with the I.P., whether it is the acting-out kid, the drinking dad, or the don't-care teen, and straighten him or her out; you'll tell the couple whether or not they should to ahead and get divorced) are not. Establishing rapport involves finding out specifically what expectations the family had in mind—"How did you hope I could help you? What do you think counseling will be like?"—and either giving them what they expect, or explaining why you can't or won't. Knowing what they're expecting is the first step in doing either.

- *Themes:* "No matter what I do, nobody in this family seems to appreciate it."

"Every time I get close to someone they leave."
"You can only depend on yourself."
"Men are only interested in themselves."
"It seems that no matter how hard I try I never quite make it."
"There's a purpose for everything, even the bad things."
"If you try hard enough, you can do anything."
"Life is just filled with pain. You just have the make the best of it."

Themes are our own private philosophy of life, our own variations of Murphy's Law, the moral of the story that is us. They are found in the larger patterns that make up our lives. They are shaped from the messages we received from parents about life, from our culture, from what we saw modeled in their own lives, from the backward glance we take when looking at our own experiences. They are often heard as the concluding sentence in a long paragraph of complaints: "I'm always waiting for the other shoe to drop"; "It's the story of my life." They can be discovered in a genogram, in a guided fantasy, or through projective testing as the same images and outcomes are repeated over and over again, or as they emerge slowly as the family begins to shed its anxiety and secrets. However they are gathered, they are powerful as summarizers of the individual's life and sense of destiny.

By hearing the themes, restating them to the family, and even challenging them, you can help families begin to see how this particular problem and possible solution fits into the larger landscape of their lives. By questioning their life assumptions, you can offer them hope that this time they can do something different, create a different outcome, and reverse the self-fulfilling prophecy. When the theme can be expressed as an image—always making it to the dock just as the boat pulls away, always reaching out your hand and having others turn away, always standing together back to back so that no one can sneak up and get you all from behind—the image can linger and come to express for the family or the individual the replication of the problem or the long-term goal to strive for.

• *Patterns of communication.* Good communication is, of course, the elementary process that binds both good family life and good therapy. Often, politely, pointing out to the family members when basic rules of communication (e.g., letting everyone speak, not interrupting, making "I" statements, talking about feelings rather than facts, etc.) are being violated is all that's needed to help the family become unstuck and begin to solve their problems on their own more effectively. In the first session facilitating good communication is often a priority and the first step in treatment.

• *Reaction to the therapist.* The reaction of the different family members to you tells you what you need to do to establish rapport. If Dad is angry and silent, you goal is to calm him down and get him talking. Generally all you need to do is explicitly say that you understand and accept his feeling angry. If Mom seems intimidated, your goal would be to get her to relax. You may want to talk about your own frustrations as a parent, or try joking with her a bit to help her see more of your humanity, rather than just your authority.

Their reaction also tells you about your perceived power and influence, and suggests ways you can use it effectively. If the parents, for example, seem extremely attentive to what you say, if they look to you as the expert or as having some magical ability to fix their child, you might wonder not only how this stance may be part of the problem (do they lack confidence as parents and see the solution as completely outside themselves?), but also whether you can use their respect for your abilities to create change more quickly. Are they more likely, for example, to try and use a behavioral chart at home that you suggest that session? Can you be more directive and they more receptive to the notion that there may be a link between their child's behavior and their tense marital relationship?

On the other hand, if your power is perceived as minimal, if you are quickly dismissed by the key members of the family, if they start off by challenging what you say or shaking their heads, look for ways to increase your power. Take more time to build rapport between you and the members of the family; clarify their expectations about therapy and your role and specifically address them; let them know about your qualifications and successes; demonstrate your expertise by providing helpful information about the problem; clarify your authority, for example, your ability to write a recommendation letter to the court or the mandate to notify social services. Make sure they are behind you before attempting to move ahead into new challenges and changes. You don't want to march ahead only to discover later that they've hung back and you're marching ahead alone.

• *Emotional range.* The ability to express a wide range of emotions is like having a full scale of notes upon which we create the melodies of our lives. For many of us, however, our range is limited, and some of us are truly one-note johnnies (e.g., I'm sad, I get angry; I'm frustrated, I get angry; I feel lonely, I get angry). Our emotional flexibility is shaped by social and cultural norms (men don't cry, women aren't supposed to get angry), and by the models we absorbed in our childhoods within the family. Often emotions are suppressed or distorted through drugs or alcohol, acted out (e.g., spending too much money, having affairs) or shrouded in an ever-present cloud of anxiety. Having a limited emotional range, like a limited verbal vocabulary, can cause others to misinterpret you or not really understand what your inner world is like.

In a family session you may see emotional range spread out among the various family members: for example, Dad only gets mad, Mom always cries, Jake is disruptive in class, or Emily gets depressed, where each relies on his or her own comfortable emotion and only together is the family able to complete the emotional scale. Often one person's designated emotion serves as a vicarious outlet for one or more of the others: Mom's easy tears express vicariously for Dad his own inexpressible deep sadness; Jake's open hostility toward his father allows Mom to vicariously express her own rage toward Dad as well; or the children's intense sibling rivalry dramatizes the parents' more subtle marital tensions. The need for and de-

pendence upon these indirect emotional outlets can be strong and difficult to give up. Even when the consequences are negative (Jake and his
father have an awful relationship), the person needing the emotional outlet will subtly reinforce them, locking the family members into unhealthy
patterns.

Simply asking who feels what or observing the process will tell you
what's missing in each person's emotional life, and in what ways the
emotional range of each individual needs to expand. Your next step may
then be to close off the vicarious outlets (Jake and Dad avoid fighting)
in order to enable the others to experience and label their emotions directly.

All this wading into new emotions can raise everyone's anxiety, including your own. As new emotions begin to bubble up, the family's reaction will be to ignore, criticize, or analyze them to death. What these new
emotional sprouts need most is recognition, space, nurturance by you.
Resist your own inclination to dampen the process or jump too quickly
toward heady solutions and new behaviors. Instead let the others know
that's it okay, that they don't need to be afraid of Mom's outburst or Dad's
tears. Model good listening, waiting, compassion, and positive feedback
for taking the risk. By once again demonstrating the simple courage of
moving against your own grain, you help the family see what new experiences can emerge.

Much of the information about these questions will come from simple observation and listening; what is left, you can ask about directly.
Taken all together they form a foundation for developing and confirming
your own initial hypothesis and setting treatment goals. In the next chapter we look at the specific goals of these opening sessions.

Looking Within: Chapter 5 Exercises

1. What are the themes in your own life? As you look back at your
past and patterns, what is the moral of your own life story so far?
How is it different or similar to that of your family? How do you
think it influences your work with others?

2. If you have had personal experience with therapy, try and re-member your own expectations, particularly of those first couple of sessions. If you have not, what would you look for most?

3. What is your own emotional range? What emotions do have dif-ficulty recognizing in yourself? Are there certain emotions that you depend on others to express for you? Practice increasing your awareness of those less familiar emotions.

4. Some people naturally talk more or less than others. In order to increase your own verbal flexibility, try experimenting in per-sonal relationships with going against your own grain and see what happens.

[6]

Great Beginnings II

THE FIRST-SESSION FLOW

There's no blueprint that will tell you how to handle a first session—what happens will depend upon the people, the problem, and your own style. But there are objectives to aim for and a way of thinking about the first session that can make it more manageable. A good first session is like a movement of a symphony or a well-written essay: There's an opening, the statement of the theme or problem, variations and development, a return to the opening theme, and closure, with each part connected to the one before. To make this all easier to follow, it may help to move through stages of the session sequentially.

1. The Preview

This is the information you get prior to the initial session. It may be the intake staff's three-sentence note based on a phone contact with one of the family members that states the problem and its history, along with a demographic checklist form, or it may be your own phone conversation with a family. Whatever the source, this information is generally minimal, often blaming, but usually enough to get your wheels turning, and give you ideas for developing an initial hypothesis.

Suppose, for example, you received the intake sheet for the Adamsons: "Boys fighting a lot; Daniel recently caught breaking into a house. Parents self-referred." Even with this minimum of information you can begin to brainstorm areas for exploration: the ways the parents discipline the children, any precipitating factors, whether the courts are involved, the way anger is handled within the family, and so on. The self-referral could be taken as saying something positive about their motivation or their desperation.

You can also decide who you want to see at that first session. Some clinicians in cases like this prefer to see the parents alone first. This gives them an opportunity to gather all the background information they need, allows them to explore the couple's ability to form a united front as well as assess the marital relationship, bond with them (they are paying the bill, after all) and talk about strategies they can begin to implement right away. Others prefer to see the entire family as a unit in action from the start and connect with everyone at the same time. Sometimes the parents themselves have strong preferences ("I think it would be good for me and my husband to give you some background"), or they can tell you what they feel may work the best ("Yes, I think Sue might feel ganged up on and say nothing if it's just the three of us and you; I can bring in the other kids"). It's a question of style, skill, and clinical thinking.[1] I suggest bringing in as many people as your anxiety and skill can manage, to help you gather the most important information you need. Once you're warmed up and have a better idea what's going on, invite the family dog and anyone else who's left or important.

2. The Opening

Armed with these preliminary ideas and your knowledge of what to avoid, you're ready to see the family. You meet them in the waiting room, lead them to your office, make sure everyone has a seat. A brief introduction—how formal or descriptive depends on your own style, the need to match the style and culture of the family, and your own sense of how much formality or information will help or hurt rapport (e.g., if you see them eyeing your degrees hanging on the wall, you might want to mention something about your background). Giving them a chance to ask questions

---

[1]Speaking of style and clinical thinking, Carl Whitaker, one of the grandfathers of family therapy, always insisted that the entire family come to the first session, no compromises. He felt that the therapist needed to win this "battle over structure" as a way of getting the therapy off on the right foot. See Augustus Napier, *The Family Crucible*, Harper Collins, 1988, for a great description of this approach.

about you models openness and helps them feel that they are not the only ones on the hot seat.

Shift to small talk. "Allen, where do you work?" "Terry, what's it like to teach third grade?" "Brian, do you play soccer?" "Daniel, do you like the new gym teacher at your school?" Or, to a small child, "What's your best friend's name?" This beginning can involve one question per person, or a brief chat with each one. This is connecting—part of building rapport, part of assessing the anxiety of each person as well as his or her ability and willingness to talk, to participate spontaneously and stray beyond your question, to express his or her attitude toward you. But whatever you say, by talking first you're helping the family to hear and get used to your voice, allowing them to settle down and get oriented before they have to talk about themselves. There's a fine line here, of course, between establishing rapport, calming everyone down, and procrastinating in order to avoid your own anxiety; make small talk too long and they'll begin to feel like you are wasting their time. Once everyone seems settled, move on.

3. Tell Me Why You're Here

Time to go to work. "Did you all talk about coming here today?" Often they haven't, and one or all of the children will shake their heads or shrug. Turning to the parents you ask, "Why don't you tell the children why you all are here?" Notice who speaks up, whether the parents are in agreement or contradict each other. If they have discussed this at home, ask if someone can summarize what was said. While older children know about counselors from school, young children may not, and if the parents mention doctor, you may need to reassure them that you don't give shots—instead tell them that you help people with worries. What you want from this opening is a clear definition of the problem and an understanding by everyone of why they are there.

All this becomes the start for a larger exploration and discussion of problems and process in the family: "What do you think about what your mom just said?" "Allen, do you feel as worried about this as your wife?" "Annie, what are you most worried will happen if things keep going the way they have?" Don't let any one person do all the talking; check in with everyone about their view of what's going on. Daniel, for example, may tell his version of the break-in, or the boys may start to argue right there in the room, demonstrating the problem the parents are describing.

Watch what the parents do, but don't let it go on and on; remember, you don't want to replicate the problem too long.

If everyone talks in vague and general terms ("He gets in trouble"; "The boys just don't mind"), get the speaker to be more specific ("How does Brian get in trouble?" "What do they do when you ask the boys to do something?"). Specificity not only helps you begin to map out patterns, and gives everyone else a better picture of behaviors involved, but helps to draw out the emotions that are masked by murky language.

The process goal is to get everyone talking, and talking more openly about things that are difficult. Be careful of setting up a pattern of asking questions and everyone giving one word answers (children, especially, will mimic their parents) or waiting for you to ask the next one. You want to encourage interaction as long as it isn't destructive, and can generally do so by looking down and not interrupting. You may need to pull in the silent ones or gently restrain the domineering ones. This gives everyone a sense that you are in charge and able to control what is happening so that it is safe enough to speak.

After you understand the presenting problems, the next shift is to the family's theory. "So, Allen and Terry, why do you think the boys have been fighting so much?" or "Why do you think Daniel broke into the house with the other boys?" Again, listen for agreement or dissension among the parents, listen to what the boys have to say, see how useful their theories are in approaching the problem—for example, "Daniel is just an angry boy [implied: like his father] who always starts the fight and gets into trouble" (possible scapegoat theory with Daniel needing to be fixed), versus "We think the boys act up when there's tension between us" (parents thinking systemically with willingness to deal with marital relationship) versus "This seemed to have started when their grandfather died" or " . . . since Daniel starting hanging out with that group of kids from the high school (unresolved family loss, influence of peers that parents feel little control over). From the theory comes what the family members have done to try solving the problem—used time-outs, ignored, yelled, tried to work on the marital relationship, tried to be nice, and so on. Look for consistency, agreement, what works, who enacts, and who enforces.

Use your questions to track where the solution breaks down: Often family members are on the right track but give up too quickly or don't know when to back off; if their solution has the potential to work (and is not illegal), you can build on it and their strengths. "What do you do when he won't go to his room?" for example. Get a clear sense of the pattern—"I yell; he refuses; I call Allen; he pushes Brian into the room; Brian runs out; we give up"—and why it occurs. If it seems appropriate at the conclusion of this discussion, ask how they specifically see therapy helping to do something different.

4. Explore

Once you have mapped out the ground around the presenting problem, it's time to go exploring. I tend to imagine the presenting problem as a large stone or wall sitting in the middle of field. What you're doing during this stage is walking around the field, exploring all the surrounding area. This is like putting an excerpt of a story in a larger context. Now you want to gather the information you need to build or confirm your hypothesis based upon your theory. For example, you may ask Allen and Terry how they go about making decisions in general, or about their own childhoods and upbringing; you may ask everyone about the death of the grandfather a year ago.

While you listen to their answers you're studying the process—the family's ability to communicate, the ability of the couple to give and take, when and with whom the children take sides. As you raise questions about a broader range of topics beyond the presenting problem (e.g., the past, death, sex, anger), you're expanding the boundaries of therapy beyond the family's initial expectations. Even if some of the questions or topics may seem irrelevant to them at this time, you're doing something important in letting everyone know that all these subjects are comfortable enough for you and are open to future discussion. What's more, you and they begin to realize that their lives are more complicated than the fraction they talk about, maybe even more than the fraction they think about.

What you're looking for is where the energy, and with it the motivation, most easily goes. Explore their emotions and emotional range. What does each person do when he or she gets angry? When he or she feels hurt? (Often anger masks hurt; hurt can mask anger; a "don't care" stance can mask both.) Ask about loneliness, depression, what one person misunderstands most about another. Ask about their biggest worry, what they are most afraid of. Most people will easily respond to such questions.

You're stirring the pot, uncovering places where the family secrets and treasures are buried, showing how two people can feel the same but act differently.

You are also discovering how well the family can follow your lead. Do they make the effort to honestly answer your questions, or do they provide only a vague answer and drift back to their own comfort zone of topics and focus? You want to continue to build rapport, yet you want to continue to move them toward their anxiety. Use questions, like a spade, to cut into new ground and raise anxiety; use comments, like a rake, to support, smooth over, and reduce it. Create a balance between the two, as well as between your talking and their talking. If you feel like you are getting stuck or pulling teeth, go back to the process in the room and talk about getting stuck or pulling teeth.

5. Create an Experience

In the best of all possible first sessions you would like to create out of your exploration an opportunity for the family to experience their process in a dramatically different way. It's actually not too difficult to do if you avoid replicating the problem and process, block, interrupt, or disrupt the dysfunctional patterns and explore outside the comfortable range of the presenting problem.

One of the simplest ways of creating such an experience comes from the tapping of new emotions. Basically you want to ask questions that give voice to the emotions that you suspect lie below the surface, that show the other side of a person, and track them until they are revealed. For example, you may ask Daniel if he misses his grandfather; move toward specificity and ask him what he remembers most about him; ask what they said to each other the last time they met. The content itself is less important than its use as a medium to stir the emotions connected to his grief.

Similarly, you may gently ask Terry, who always seems to be yelling at Daniel, to describe how she felt when Daniel was born, what her hopes are for his future, or how she felt when her mother used to scold her— questions that lead Terry to express that softer side of herself and change the emotional climate in the room. When this type of probing is successful it creates some of the most powerful of experiences because they seem to catch everyone by surprise. New emotions come to the surface that are rarely expressed by that person or within the family.

You can also create an experience through *enactments*. In order to be successful, they require some staging. Focus on a specific topic that two family members have had trouble discussing, and which both have something to gain by talking about it. Ask Dad and Brian, for example, to talk there about Brian's push for a larger allowance—what he wants, what Dad expects, if anything, in the way of responsibilities. Have the two brothers see if they can come up with a plan for sharing game time on the computer. Be clear about what they should try and accomplish, and interrupt only to keep the conversation going, not to preach. You'll know by their awkwardness and hesitation whether everyone is going against their emotional and behavioral grain. The outcome not only tells you not only about their ability to try something new, but unlocks new emotions as the behaviors holding them are broken.[2]

You can, if the family seems open and engaged, also stage an experiential event. For example, have them create a family sculpture: Have everyone stand up, and ask the I.P. (or have several family numbers take turns) to create a sculpture of the family as he or she sees it, without using words. Place everyone in a physical position that represents how he or she seems to be most of the time (Mom is scowling and shaking her finger, Dad is off in the corner reading the paper), located where each one most often seems to be (Mom is next to Sis, Dad is way off in the corner by himself), making sure the sculptor is included. Ask them to change the sculpture to create their view of the ideal family (Mom and Dad are holding hands, with the kids in-between). By working the image (Dad, how does it feel out there all by yourself? Mom, what facial expression do you see yourself having most of the time?) you create images that you can manipulate and work with later. Emotionally, these can be powerful.

Finally, you can create experience through interpretation and insight: Talk to Dad, for example, about his own childhood, and point out how his own reaction to Daniel's behavior is exactly what he just said he hated in his own father; mention to the couple how the patterns of their own arguments so well mimic those of the boys, or how the boys' struggles over the computer are similar to their own tensions about individual versus couple time; help Brian acknowledge that though he really wants his dad's attention, his misbehavior doesn't work, and actually only makes

[2]For more information on enactments see Salvador Minuchin, *Family Therapy Techniques*, Harvard University Press, 2004.

matters worse. The insight is always in the eyes of the beholder; it is not an insight not because it seems clever to you or is accurate in content, but because of the emotional impact it has on the listener.

Creating an experience, however it is achieved, gives the family a fuller sense of what therapy is like, that it can be more than the talking they have already done at home. It increases intimacy and rapport, enhances your credibility, and gives you a sense of what possibly works with this particular family.

6. Go Back to the Problem

You can't simply stir up emotions and leave them. This will only make the some family members fearful of therapy process and of you as the therapist; others will feel anxious simply because they don't know where this is all leading. Once again explanation follows experience. You have to ground the experience by linking it and the exploration back to their initial concern. Now that you have explored the area in the field around the stone, you have to return back to it.

This is where you lay out your hypothesis for the family: "I know you both think that the housebreaking has something to do with the boys Daniel was playing with, but, Daniel, it seems like you are still pretty sad about your grandfather; I wonder if those feelings are connected to the hard time you have been having lately." Or, "Terry, it seems like it's easy for you to get angry, and the boys have been doing a pretty good job of keeping you stirred up, but I also can see that underneath this anger is a lot of worry and concern and caring that the boys rarely get to see." Or, "Allen, it seems like you have been doing your best over the years to not be abusive toward your children like your father was with you. But it seems that even though you are able to ignore the boys' behavior for a long periods of time, it only makes matters worst; eventually you blow up, scaring the boys and confirming the fear that you were trying to avoid."

What you are doing is giving the family a new theory to replace the old one, showing them how the presenting problems are poor solutions, how their ability to solve the problem is undermined by other problems and emotions that are they are not seeing. This gives the family a new perspective, and with that a new energy and a new way of tackling the problem—Daniel isn't a bad kid, but a kid who is unable to express his grief; Allen isn't screwing up, he's struggling to overcome the modeling he received from his own father; Terry isn't a mean witch, but someone who has developed a tough side and is having difficulty letting others know how she really feels or needs.

Having said that, you need to know whether your idea flies, especially with those who hold the most power in the family. Ask each one for his or her reaction. Look for the subtle shaking of the head, the quiet but clear "yes, but," the tacit agreement with little enthusiasm. It's important that your idea becomes their own or they won't be motivated to follow you further. Unless Allen makes the connection among the boys, him, and his own father, unless Terry can agree that her more comfortable anger is blocking her expression of concern and distorting her relationship with her sons, unless both of them and Daniel believe that there truly is a link between the grief and his acting out, you have no foundation on which to built a therapeutic contract. But if the rapport is there, if they feel as though you listened and understood their concern, if the experience was powerful enough to shake up their assumptions without overwhelming them, they will agree with your point of view. If there is resistance to your ideas, fix the problem in the room, confront them, talk about the process: "Terry, you're shaking your head; it seems like you don't see it the same way I am; what are you thinking?" Listen carefully to what the client says, see where the snags are, use education to help connect the dots.

7. Set Goals, Describe Your Plan

If everyone is on the same page, move ahead. Suggest the next steps: "I'd like to spend some time with you by yourself next time, Daniel, if you and your parents don't mind, to talk some more about how you've been feeling"; "Maybe it would be good if you both could try and switch roles; maybe you, Allen, could take over the disciplining so that Terry can have a chance to get out of being the bad guy. Why don't you both come by yourselves next time and we can talk about it."

All this doesn't mean that you need to have everything worked out in 50 minutes. If you still need more information, if you need to spend more time getting to know one of the family members better, just say so. Be honest about what you are thinking and where you stand: "I'm wondering how much this is all connected to the recent loss of your grandfather. Would you be willing to meet and talk more about this next week?" "I know I've been talking a lot to your parents today; could I talk to you guys by yourselves next time?" "I think I can help you with setting up clearer rules at home, but I'd like to do some psychological testing first." Being clear and specific about both what you need and how you'd like to go about getting it reduces the family's anxiety and gives them a sense of movement and direction.

8. Homework and Closure

Homework is valuable for several reasons. It lets the family know that therapy isn't just talking about things for an hour in a room, but working and making changes in their daily lives as well. It keeps the momentum created in the session going. Most importantly it gives you a test of the family's motivation in regard to both your direction and their willingness to make changes at home. It shows you what works and doesn't work (e.g., the behavioral chart was too complicated), and where in specific ways the change process breaks down (Mom gives in if the child tantrums in a public place). Describe the homework to the family not as a solution to the problem, but rather as an experiment to try and to see what happens. When they come back next time, you can all use it as a starting point for beginning the session.

You might ask Terry, for example, to track those times when she begins to feels angry by sitting down for a minute and asking herself what she's worried about. You could ask Allen what his father remembers about Allen's childhood or about his father's own childhood. You could challenge the boys to see if they could discover other, more positive ways (rather than fighting) to snag their parent's attention during the week, and see what works the best.

The homework needn't be elaborate—it can be as simple as the parents contacting the school and getting a copy of the test results, the couple coming up together with a list of questions they want to discuss next week, asking a mother and daughter to have a five-minute discussion on what was good during the day, or suggesting that the father try and resist the temptation to leave the house when he starts to get mad. All it needs to be is something that helps the family link the session process with their real lives, and this initial session with the next.

Closing the session—shifting briefly back to small talk, perhaps, shaking hands once again, thanking them for coming, walking them out—serves as a ritual that provides a symmetry to the session, and helps to ease the transition back to the outside world.

Once again, all these suggestions are not a blueprint for what you have to do, but a way of describing the overall session structure, flow, and balance. If you keep this in mind together with the basics, the session will move in the direction you want it to go.

THE SECOND SESSION

Some therapists do reminder calls to families between sessions. Doctors, dentists, even hair stylists now do this routinely, calling and leaving a message reminding the family of the time of the next appointment a day or so before. It can reduce cancellations or blank spaces in your appointment schedule, and many families have come to expect it. But it is time consuming, especially if you have to do it yourself, and some therapists object on philosophical grounds—clients should take responsibility for their obligations, and/or the therapist feels like a parent reminding Maggie that she needs to clean up her room before going to the mall.

While it can seem like a courtesy service, and I personally have been fine with it when it was routinely done by support staff in an agency setting (I always asked the family if they minded such a call before the end of the first session), I've tended not to do this in my one-man private practice for several reasons: It is a time issue; I do assume families can be responsible; it does feel a bit intrusive (Can I leave messages on the house answering machine or is that a problem?); and I'm also clear about my cancellation policy at the beginning. There have been a few exceptions—when clients may genuinely struggle with following a schedule, such as when there are issues of mental retardation or when they may be emotionally overwhelmed for few weeks, or when I find that I'm not clear, for whatever reason, about the next appointment time—but these are rare. Like most other decisions we have been talking about, I believe it's best not to be arbitrary or base your decision on what was done at your last job or what your colleagues do. Think it through, and be clear about your reasons and motivations so the family understands them as well.

Whatever you decide, the second session feels different than the first. Those first-session butterflies are gone and everyone feels more settled, but the family is not yet likely to be ready to take over major responsibility for the process. You need to have specific goals and start things off. What do you need to do in this session? Here are several options:

• *Finish up what's left over from the last session.* Is there someone in family that you need to meet—the grandmother, the older brother who was working last time, the father who was out of town on a business trip? Is there someone who you need to get to know better, someone who didn't quite connect with you—the little sister who spent the last session playing with the blocks in the corner, the father who nodded his head and said the right things but seemed to be only half listening and minimally involved, the I.P., who, in spite of your efforts, may still have felt beaten up by everyone else and who needs to see that you can be an advocate for him or her as well? Is there additional information that you need—a better assessment of the mother's depression, a history of the father's past addiction, a clearer picture of just what it is that the parents do when the kids refuse to go to bed, a better sense of just how much the little girl is affected by all the fighting?

It's in this second session that you may wish to pull the family apart (or bring them all together if you decided to only see part of the group before)—for example, seeing one of the parents individually if you felt he or she was holding back for some reason last time, doing play therapy with one of the children to build rapport and to get a better idea of his or her world, talking to the siblings without the parents to see how they act differently. These are ways of further defining goals and establishing contact and contracts with various family members, narrowing problems, or determining where the energy and motivation most lie.

If you decide to split up the family, make sure no one feels left out or paranoid about what's going on. Tell the parents why you want to see the boys by themselves so that they don't imagine that you're going to be pumping them to reveal the family's secrets. If you see one child, spend at least a few minutes with the others, so that they don't feel excluded and that you don't reinforce the notion that only that child has problems. If you see an adult alone, balance it out either by then seeing the other, or by seeing the couple and having the individual explain what you both had discussed.

Similarly, avoid talking about someone behind his or her back. Don't be fooled into thinking that what you think you may say to one "in confidence" isn't likely to get repeated to the others. Not only does saying to a wife that it seems to you that her husband has trouble with intimacy or is depressed border on being unethical, it clinically unbalances the relationship among you, the husband, and the wife. You're treating the husband as though he were a child, and setting up a potential opportunity for the wife to use this against her husband outside the office. Similarly, telling a brother that his sister is probably jealous of him is often a surefire way to have the sister find out that you are saying what you think about her behind her back and for it to undermine your relationship with her.

• *Firm up your diagnosis for the I.P.* Even the most purist of family therapists in an agency or in private practice is required to provide a *Diagnostic and Statistical Manual of Mental Disorders* (DSM) diagnosis on one member of the family for funding, charting, or managed care requirements. If you weren't able to do this after the first session, now is the time. Most often when a child or teen is identified by the parents as having the "problem," it is usually around him or her that the chart is built and the diagnosis assigned. What you think about diagnoses and how you use them will depend upon your theory, philosophy, and style. Some therapists begin and end with viewing problems in traditional family therapy terms, with individual diagnosis as secondary and supplemental— something they just need to do and get done for paperwork reasons, or as a statement of individual concerns that usually can be addressed in family process. Others lean toward the other pole, clinically giving more weight to diagnosis from the beginning; they build upon it, and look upon family therapy as the means for best addressing the behaviors and symptoms it represents.

My own view is that an individual diagnosis is really a matter of balancing out individual and family process. While some diagnoses like depression, psychosis, addictions, and obsessive–compulsive disorder (OCD) require assessing individual treatment needs from the start (medication for depression or psychosis, specialized addiction treatment, individual cognitive-behavioral therapy for OCD), others do not—for example, oppositional defiant disorder or conduct disorder in children and teens. If the individual's symptoms interfere with his or her ability to effectively use family therapy (e.g., symptoms of major depression or psychosis interfere with the ability to effectively interact within a family session), then addressing these individual concerns at the beginning makes sense. But I still want to ask myself the same questions I ask of any family: How does this behavior fit within the context of the family? How can I give the family a new way of looking at the problem (e.g., does focusing on the child's attention-deficit/hyperactivity disorders [ADHD] give the parents a new, more compassionate way of seeing their child or only reinforce his or her role as the problem?) What is the family's own expectation and motivation for family treatment? What impact will changes within the family system have on the individual's behaviors and symptoms?

The answers to these questions will determine how the individual diagnosis will fit into the larger treatment plan. What I know I don't want to do is have the family look upon a diagnosis as a way of "patientizing" the family member or use it as a rationale for scapegoating, not looking at or taking responsibility for the larger family process.

• *Find out more about what works.* This is where you ask about the homework, either in your small groups or all together. Simply by asking about their experience with the homework gives the family the message that you take homework seriously and that you expect them to do it. If they didn't, ask them to explain why—for example, "I mentioned it to Kadrian but he just shrugged and I didn't press it"; "John had to suddenly go out of town for four days"; "We started to, but realized we didn't really understand what to do." If these seem like limp excuses, probe a bit further: Were they feeling too anxious about doing it, were they worried about doing it wrong, does it reflect something about their attitude toward you, the therapy, or your initial assessment of the problem?

Pinning this down tells you where the obstacles lie and what you need to do to remove them. You may discover that you were moving too fast, asking them to do more than they could emotionally handle, or didn't do a good enough job is selling your theory, leaving one of the key people unconvinced and uncooperative. Or perhaps the family's response only replicated the way they respond to other problems, challenges, or pressure from the outside, namely, by ignoring them.

If they did the homework, you want to know what they thought about it. Sometimes the family will do exactly what you ask, and the assignment will accomplish exactly what you behaviorally hoped it would, but the results seem to have little emotional impact on the family: Sure, Dad spent more time with Brian and they had a good time, but Dad says it wasn't much different than the times he'd done it before, and he seems unimpressed. Perhaps Dad doesn't see the connection of the assignment to his concerns, doesn't understand your assessment of the problem, or isn't aligned with you and therapy and is merely going through the motions. If the assignment was tried but didn't work, that is, the family wasn't able to carry it out (Mom still got mad, Brian still was fighting) you want to track where it broke down so you can help the family fine-tune it, or rethink your hypothesis.

It's also a good idea at this session to ask what they thought about the last one. Not only may you find out what someone didn't like ("I felt you were taking Allen's side") or what made them uncomfortable ("I was surprised how hard it was to talk to Brian about his schoolwork"), but also what, of all that went on, had the largest impact on specific individuals ("What you said about my father really got me thinking"; "Having a chance to hear what Terry really thought was helpful"; "Feeling that it wasn't all my fault helped me be less critical of myself") clues to what you may want to use again. Even if they say little in response to your question, by asking the question you are letting them know that their feedback about the therapy process is welcomed.

• *Help the family further understand how the therapy process will work.* If you ask how their week was, or what problems came up, they quickly assume that the therapy will include monitoring on a week-by-week process. If, on the other hand, you take a less directive role and ask the couple or family what they want to talk about, or continue to explore their past, the family will begin to think that this is what the meetings will be like.

Because they look to you to set the pace, be deliberate in what you're doing. Once again the best route to take is one of creating balance, between initiating and responding, the individual and the group, assessment and treatment. Back up your actions with clear communication: "I know I've been asking a lot of question during these two sessions; next time I won't be; I'd like you to think about what we need to talk about and bring it up." "We're going to complete the psychological testing these next two weeks, then I'll come back to you with the results and some suggestions." Let them know how you are thinking so they can begin to do the same.

THE TOP SIX FAMILY STRUCTURES

By the end of this second session, you should feel more certain about your hypothesis, feel more connected to everyone in the family, have gathered the missing information that you needed or know what is left to get, and have an idea of what works. Here are some of the most common family presentations and structures to look for, along with their overall goals, and the pitfalls to avoid:

1. The "Fix My Child" Parents

Characteristics: Parents present a united picture of the identified child as the cause and solution of his or her own and the family's problems.

Goals: Engage with parents by initially talking to them in the language of the child's problem (e.g., What do you do when Frank gives you a hard time?); assess child; help parents see the child's behavior in a new light (e.g., educate them about ADHD) or as the outcome of larger family process; find out what the parents disagree about; empower parents to be change agents within the family.

What not to do: Do only individual therapy with child beyond the initial assessment.

2. The Enmeshed versus Disengaged Parents

Characteristics: In these families one parent, often the mother, is overly involved with the children, is supportive, and has difficulty setting structure or limits—that is, the parent is enmeshed. The other parent, usually the father, seems distant and aloof, acts as the disciplinarian, and struggles to be supportive—that is, this parent is disengaged and distant. He usually gets pulled in by Mom when she is overwhelmed by the behavior of the children, or steps in when he feels she is being too soft.

Goals: Bring Father into therapy process; help parents see how their differences are creating problems; work toward improving their relationship and creating a united front; have Father support Mother in being more powerful rather than continuing to take over limit setting.

What not to do: Re-create the structure in therapy, that is, ignore Father, re-create the Father's role as limit-setter of children in session and leave Mother unempowered; polarize with Mother over how to best manage the children.

3. The Overwhelmed Single Parent

Characteristics: Chaotic family, little structure or consistency, often a history of abuse.

Goals: Empower parent through skill building, encouragement; support parent to get through emotional stuck-points; divide problems into more manageable segments; help reduce environmental stressors.

What not to do: Take over and rescue parent; create unreasonable dependency upon you; become overwhelmed yourself.

4. The Crisis Family

Characteristics: Family easily feels victimized by life events, takes a reactive stance to problems, often has an "us versus the world" mind-set.

Goals: Build trust by initially encouraging family to contact you when in crisis; help family move from the black/white of crisis/no problem by recognizing early signs of problems and taking action.

What not to do: Work harder than the family; create too strong a dependency by maintaining the on-call rescuer role for crises; be reactive in your own behavior and wind up feeling in crisis yourself.

5. The Transitional Family

Characteristics: Essentially a combination of the dynamics of the enmeshed/disengaged parents and the overwhelmed single parent. Disciplinarian leaves the family; the remaining parent is unable to set structure; one of children steps up to replace missing the parent, then feels entitled and may even be abusive toward the remaining parent.

Goals: Develop limit-setting and structure-setting skills in parent; facilitate grief over lost parent; help entitled child find new, healthier role within family.

What not to do: Replace the missing parent's role.

6. The Referred/No-Problem Family

Characteristics: Another agency defines the problem, mandates therapy; the family is openly angry or passive-aggressive.

Goals: Be clear about role; have referral source clarify concerns; explore treatment options and consequences; find a problem/goal that the family is willing to work on.

What not to do: Be the enforcer for the referring agency.

Obviously you will find variations on these common structures, and I talk about some of them later in more detail. Again, what is important is both meeting expectations and reshaping them, moving toward what's missing, and avoiding replicating the problem.

THIRD-SESSION SHIFT,
OR HOW DID I LOSE THEM?

Generally by the third session things have settled down—your assessment is complete or nearly complete, rapport is high and the family feels comfortable with you, expectations are clear, and the treatment process is turning the corner toward the start of the middle phase. But not always. Sometimes the third session slides out from beneath you—the family gets ornery, maybe even quits, or everyone, including you, suddenly seems to run out of steam, all catching you off guard. Here are some of what might be going on underneath the third-session shift:

• Families in crisis or who are crisis-oriented may have calmed down simply by telling their stories and hearing your suggestions, or because outside events have changed (e.g., the dad found a new job, the school is not going to press charges). They don't see the need to continue and simply drop out, or they are exhausted from expending all their energy on the crisis. They may have difficulty understanding the underlying issues, or doing the preventative work that can keep the next crisis from brewing altogether.

As mentioned earlier, if you suspect the family functions this way, educating them about crisis reactions and the possible recurrence of the problem can be useful; help them emotionally see the connection between underlying issues and surface behavior. If they are still wary, offer them an appointment to come back for a checkup in a few weeks or months to encourage a preventive, proactive stance rather than a reactive one, or ask them if they mind if you give them a call just to check and see how they are doing.

But if they are set on leaving, let them do so with your support. Unless you have clear clinical reservations—the son still seems extremely depressed and potentially suicidal—let them leave feeling good about themselves, rather than with the message and guilt from you that you think they're failing to follow through. If they feel supported in leaving, they will feel supported in coming back.

- Similarly, some families take two or more sessions to ventilate and get things off their chests, and then get anxious. They look up and realize that you're in the room with them and panic over what they think you think; they wonder what might happen next. One way to handle this is to anticipate it: Talk about the process, give voice to their feelings, map out the logical next step.

- After a couple of sessions countertransference and transference begin to settle in. The parents decide that you are not as all-knowing as they originally thought, the mother realizes that she really does have a hard time talking openly with men, you begin to feel that the family is not as motivated as you initially believed. They close up or drop out; you start acting more pushy. Talk to your supervisor to help you from overreacting. Talk about what you see: "It feels like we were going strong for a few weeks, but now we're slowing down"; educate them about and normalize the process ("Most families in counseling feel most enthusiastic the first few weeks, then they begin to feel that they are not making as much progress"); help them sort through their feelings ("Terry, you seem annoyed about what I've been suggesting") to keep these emotions from replicating the family process and undermining the therapy.

- If you see only a portion of the family the first time or two (e.g., the mother or father isn't able to come), the missing ones may feel left out of the process, or resist coming in and sabotage it for everyone else, causing them all to drop out. In couple therapy this often takes the form of the wife coming in first, then her telling her husband that she saw a marital therapist, who now wants to see him with her. Out of his anxiety he promises to make all the changes in the world and convinces the wife to discontinue. Seeing everyone together as soon as possible; reaching out to the missing person, even by telephone; or predicting this process for those attending and coaching them on how to respond to the other can often prevent this.

- "Fix My Child" parents are comfortable while the child is being discussed or evaluated, but may panic when you shift to larger family issues, the marriage, or themselves as individuals. As mentioned earlier, the key in these cases is pacing—meeting their initial expectations, carefully monitoring their anxiety, and making sure that you connect these larger issues to the child's presenting problem.

• Mandated families may come for the first couple of sessions, long enough for you to say that you saw them or for them to say that they came, then drop out basically because they don't want to be there. Contacting the referring agency right away and deciding with them how they want things to be handled if the family doesn't continue to come can help clarify your role, and provide a united front to the family.

Except for mandated cases, the driving force behind all these third-session shifts is anxiety, created by the shift in focus from the presenting, surface, external crisis orientation to the underlying, internal, right-now process. If you move too quickly or push to hard for them to focus on what seems too threatening, they will drop out. Maintain openness and honesty, focus on the process and make it as representative as possible of the way therapy will be, move quickly enough for the client to feel that something is happening, but not so quickly that the family feels pushed into something they don't agree with.

Periodically reiterate the treatment contract: "I think that's it's good that you came in; I think the basic problem is . . . and I think I can help; I don't think therapy needs to be a long time if we work together." Remember, you have constant feedback right there in the room. If ever you are uncertain where the family stands, ask.

When some families don't show up, therapists are often relieved. If you find all kinds of reasons not to follow up with the family, it probably says something about your own countertransference in this particular case. Generally it's a good idea to write a note or make a phone call, guessing how they may be feeling, why they may be disappointed in treatment, and inviting them to come back and talk about it. But even doing that you'll find, as was said in the first chapter, despite your good efforts, there's still much that will be beyond your control: expectations that the family simply won't reveal, individual emotional triggers or pressures on the family's life that makes them decide that therapy with you or therapy at all is no longer needed. You can only do what you are capable of doing.

The challenges of the beginning are the challenges that come with starting any joint enterprise, namely, reaching an understanding and agreement about the nature of the relationship, about the way time together will be spent and how it all will work, that is, creating a shared vision. It's a time when the rhythm of the therapy hasn't yet taken over, and you are forced to rely more on your own personal strengths. But if you can succeed in accomplishing the goals you set out for these initial sessions, most of the hard part is over. You're ready to move on to the next stage.

Looking Within: Chapter 6 Exercises

These exercises are designed to help you increase your self-awareness of the issues surrounding beginnings and to increase your observation skills by practicing them outside of therapy. Go ahead, try them over the next week.

1. Think again about your own theory, values, and personal level of anxiety. What are your greatest strengths? Who do you feel it is most important to see in the initial session? Who would you not want or feel comfortable seeing (e.g., small children, extended family)? What would help you most in reducing your own anxiety? See if you can develop in advance your rules of thumb for first sessions that would work best for you and the families you work with.

2. Rapport: We all vary in our natural sociability and outgoingness. If this initial connecting with families is awkward for you, try improving your skills in less pressured situations—meeting someone at a party, talking to the person next to you on a bus or standing in line. Increase your risk taking and comfort in connecting with a wider range of people.

3. Themes, again. Hearing themes is a matter of floating along the top of a conversation, avoiding diving down and getting stuck in the details of the content, making yourself listen for metaphoric connections, repeated phrases and images, recurring patterns. It takes practice do develop this skill. Practice listening for themes in your nonclinical conversations with friends, neighbors, family. You'll know if you are on target simply but restating the theme back to the person and seeing if it resonates for him or her.

4. Think of something that someone in your family—nuclear or family of origin—does that particularly bothers you. Write it down and describe it fully. Then consider in what ways other people in the family may be involved in provoking or maintaining this problem. For example, your father may drive fast partly because your mother is timid or is always telling him to slow down. Your spouse may seem always to overreact to one of your children because you seem to him or her to underreact or side with your child. Next try adapting the attitude that it is not about you at all, but the other person's way of seeing the world or way of coping with some emotion inside him or her. See how these new perceptions affect your feelings.

[7]

The Middle Stage

ARE WE THERE YET?

Once you've crossed over the mountains of the beginning stage, you come to the broad, flat prairie land of the middle. There's a sigh of relief for making it through those initial challenges, and you look forward to the steady rolling progress that the middle stage seems to promise. Here is where the bulk of the treatment will take place, where the visions and goals created in those first few weeks are forged into something solid and permanent.

But just as the relief starts to wane you find that for every good session or week there's one that isn't quite as good. The skills that you laboriously help the family learn—communication, parenting, assertiveness—have to be constantly relearned or fine-tuned. Just when you think all the crises are behind you, one flares up without any apparent warning. The ground, you discover, is not as flat as it seemed from the distance; the ruts and bumps you didn't see before seem at times to be all around you.

All this makes for the famous "working through" of the middle stage. The work of working through is the grind, the feeling that you are not so much a digging down deeper into the layers of the family structure and individual personalities, but rather digging a hole, filling it back up, and digging it out again. For three weeks in a row everyone does a good job of listening and sidestepping the destructive outbursts, but then Grandma shows up for a short visit and the tension causes everything to collapse back into chaos. Mom is able to hold firm on the bedtime routine, but then she has a hard day at work, the kids double-team her when Dad isn't home, and she caves in. Dad is snapping less at the kids, but still has a hair-trigger around his wife. New skills are still new and not yet integrated into the family's everyday lives. Gains are fragile, and it doesn't take much for it all to fall apart.

GETTING STUCK

While this two steps forward, one step back is probably the most common pattern seen throughout the middle stage of therapy, there are other variations. Sometimes a family will initially make progress and then not only lose ground but be back to zero within a matter of weeks.

Teresa, for example, a single parent, comes in with her two adolescent children, Lavone, age 15, and Kenisha, age 13. The presenting problems are Kenisha refusing to go to school, Lavone staying out late. In those first couple of sessions, thanks to your rapport and education, Teresa no longer is holding on to her theory that her children are bad kids made worse by their friends. She is following through on implementing the structural and behavioral changes that you both agreed upon—arranging a meeting with the school staff, herself, and Kenisha to discuss Kenisha's complaints; taking a clear, strong stand at home about the need for her to attend school regularly; setting clear limits with Lavone, and contacting the juvenile court for disciplinary backup.

It works. Kenisha goes to school for three solid weeks, and after a stern talk with the court officer, Lavone gives up testing his mother's new resolve and is staying home at night. But then everything unravels— Kenisha stays home a couple of days because she says she's sick, and it's the beginning of the end. Her excuses become thinner and thinner, and Teresa seems to lose her ability to get Teresa to school. Lavone at the same time activates the other front and stays out later and later with no consequences by Teresa. Within a month everything seems back to where it started.

What's going on here? Some of this is certainly predictable. Most families make some progress and feel great as the initial anxiety and worry are reduced. But then there's some slipup, such as Kenisha's missing of a day of school, and they become afraid—that the gains were illusory, that their original theory was right after all, that this therapy stuff really doesn't work, that they "tried" yet again and nothing changes. What they don't fully appreciate is that progress was made, not because they managed to show up in your office, but because they were beginning to do something different. They need to understand that setbacks are inevitable not because it isn't working but simply because they are inexperienced. Even after they slide back, the same skills that helped them before will help them again.

Developing behavioral consistency and holding the line in spite of one's emotional state are the real challenges at the beginning of the middle stage. To do that Teresa needs review and reinforcement of the new goals to help her stay focused, and support to take action even when she doesn't feel like it or believe she can do it. She needs help generalizing the new skills, help recognizing when seemingly new problems are really just variations on the old, and detailed coaching on what to say and do when Kenisha says she doesn't want to go to school or when Lavone comes home three hours after curfew. Most of all she needs ongoing encouragement and a pat on the back when things seem to slip.

But sometimes this skill training, reinforcement, and support are not enough. Over the weeks you find the situation to be more complicated than you originally thought; you discover other dynamics at work that weren't immediately apparent during the initial assessment. Teresa's low-grade but chronic depression, for example, her poor health, or her demanding elderly mother may sap her time and energy and make it difficult for her to keep up her on task. Other people, who originally seemed to be at the far outskirts of the family, may now appear to be more involved and undermine her efforts. Teresa's boyfriend, for example, who used work evenings, is now in the home at night, and he is jealous of the increased attention the children suddenly seem to be getting. Rather than supporting Teresa's new stance, he undermines her, urging her not to be so hard on the kids, or stands up for them when she tries to impose the new rules. If Teresa is to stay on track, she'll need your help, both concretely and emotionally, addressing these new problems that are threatening to pull her off course.

In other cases there is not so much the normal backsliding of applying new skills, or the erosion by other problems and family members, but an apparent struggle to develop real traction. There may be revolving scapegoats—for example, Kenisha isn't going to school, but Lavone is doing well, and then they switch; Kenisha seems back on track, but suddenly Lavone is talking back and slipping out at night to meet his friends on the corner—each changing emotional places and taking turns being the "good child" for a while. Other times the parent's internal process remains the same, even though she seems to be saying and doing the right things. In spite of her attempts to become firmer and more consistent, for example, you notice that Teresa still frets or yells or spends all her time consumed by the children, and gives the boyfriend cause to remain on the outskirts of the family. What these variations represent are the tenacity of the family's patterns to maintain and contain the family's emotions and roles. Rather than tackling the fundamental changes in process that are needed, anxiety pushes each of the family members toward slight shifts in focus, variations on the familiar, and prevents deeper change.

So does the sense of loss. Change implies not only the learning of new skills and roles, but often the emotional and psychological giving up of what the members of the family have for so long thought of as "life." Solving problems and breaking patterns can trigger new emotions and (as stories of lottery winners can attest) create their own new challenges. If Teresa has, for as long as she can remember, not only worried about her children but put them first, she will find her concept of herself as a mother and an adult change if her children are less of a problem and less of her focus. She will have more mental and emotional room to think about herself, raising questions, perhaps, about who is she not just as a parent, but as a person. She may have more time and energy to focus on her relationship with her boyfriend, possibly causing her to reconsider how he fits into her life, or challenging her toward new, deeper levels of intimacy. Such changes can create, a least for a while, a hole in her old identity, one that she may need to grieve and ponder before she can fill it in. This transition, grief, and challenge can run like an undertow beneath the changes going on up above and contribute to the sluggish, slowing down, plateauing feeling of the middle stage.

ANTIDOTES TO STUCKNESS

So what do you do with all this slipping, sliding, and sticking? Here are some options to consider:

• *Grind it out.* This is the modus operandi of the middle stage—plodding over the same ground again and again, keeping everyone committed and on track. This can be invaluable for the family, especially those who are crisis-oriented and never developed the skills of consistency and follow-through. They can quickly grow impatient or become distracted, and it is your perseverance that serves as a model and ultimately seeps into their thinking. Your job is to keep everyone from giving up or going of, to focus on the details in order to fine-tune the skills and strategies, and to help remove the emotional obstacles that arise (e.g., Teresa's feeling that she is being a bad mother), and to help them see how each one of them copes with the stress of change in a different way.

• *Mix it up.* Grinding it out, however, doesn't have to be deadly. The middle stage is a good time to reinforce the skills and concepts by changing formats and introducing experiential work on an irregular basis (doing it on a regular basis only flattens its potential impact). Bring in additional family members—for example, Teresa's boyfriend—see siblings together or individually, do some guided imagery, sculpt the changing family relationships. This not only helps avoid the therapeutic ruts and keeps the family interested and engaged, but helps ferret out additional problems that may undermine progress.

• *Separate/clarify problems.* Problems with children are often a more comfortable entrée into the therapy process than couple or individual ones (What parent doesn't want to help his or her child?). After a session or two focused on the children's behavior, a parent has the opportunity to see for him- or herself just how helpful or sensitive you really are before moving onto more difficult issues. Although Teresa, for example, may initially come in about Kenisha, by the second session it may become clear that it is her relationship with her boyfriend or mother that is bothering her the most. The presenting problem may be quickly resolved, sidelined, or dismissed by the family, and as the clinician you can move where the client's energy and anxiety lead you.

But sometimes it's you, not the client, who needs to do the leading. Even though Teresa is quick to dismiss her depression as just the way she has always been, it becomes apparent to you that it is undermining her ability to follow through on the suggestions you've made. A referral for a medication evaluation may be the next step needed to give her the energy to make changes and break the negative cycles, and you may need to spend some time educating and persuading her to do this. Similarly, you may feel that her relationship with her boyfriend holds the key to her acting more effectively as a parent. Your job not only becomes one of helping her see that not only are the two problems related, but that the second is actually more important. How you decide to link and prioritize this array of problems rests upon your theory and its notion of causality.

Finally, there are times when you need to decide whether a new problem is really a new problem, a variation of the old (e.g., revolving scapegoats), or a distraction. Just as families not in therapy return to comfortable problems when their anxiety and stress get too high, so too will families in therapy. This is the principle of triangulation—the reducing of anxiety and conflict between two people by both focusing instead on a more neutral issue.[1] You may notice a sudden return to old complaints, patterns, or repetition of already-told stories. As you begin to help Teresa look more closely at her relationship with her boyfriend, for example, suddenly new crises may arise at school with Kenisha or at home with Lavone, reflecting the increase in her stress that new changes are creating. If you've done a good assessment and know what are the family's comfortable problems are, you won't be led astray and can help the family discuss their anxiety and stay focused.

• *Normalize, label, diversify.* In the middle of this middle stage your role often shifts from that of a teacher educating the family to the workings of the process and new behaviors, to a that of a guide, one more familiar than they with the terrain of change. Predicting to the family the backslides, the shift in scapegoats, the eruption of crises, the feelings of anxiety and ambivalence, and the sabotage by others in the family, then normalizing the process helps them realize that they are not failing, and keeps them from feeling discouraged. It also provides the family with a sense of control as they, too, begin to understand and can anticipate just what the process of change entails.

Labeling the process has similar positive effects. For example, labeling for Teresa the school issues as her comfortable problem, the area where much of her attention and emotions so readily goes—or an adolescent's self-cutting behaviors as her way of coping when she feels emotionally overwhelmed—helps her and the rest of the family do the same. Being able to name what is happening allows the family to gain some distance, perspective, and control when these problems and emotions

---

[1]For more information on triangles and triangulation in families see Philip Guerin et al., *Working with Relationship Triangles: The One-Two-Three of Psychotherapy*, Guilford Press, 1996.

arise. The family can begin to see it as you see it, as part of the larger pattern, and are more free to approach it in a new way.

Finally, helping the family diversify their emotional outlets and expand their emotional and behavioral range by both interrupting the well-worn patterns and encouraging them to go against their own grain—helping Teresa confront her boyfriend; helping Kenisha talk to her teachers about problems, rather than cutting class—are the best ways to ensure that they have something to replace what they are giving up. Unless they each can develop greater emotional and behavioral flexibility it becomes all too easy to remain dependent and caged within the roles and patterns that they know.

• *Approach the loss.* How you handle the underlying loss that the new changes create depends both upon its power as an obstacle for the family and your own clinical and personal stance. If, for example, you are doing brief, solution-based treatment, or if the problems are not deeply ingrained, these emotions will most likely remain untouched. Rather than defining and focusing on the grief, you may simply pull the family along against its undertow until they are beyond its grasp, and the new behaviors, and the emotions they bring, take hold.

If loss is a difficult issue for you, if you are in the middle of coping with changes within your personal life, you may find yourself reluctant to tackle this topic and these emotions, and will no doubt find yourself attracted to a clinical theory that supports doing this. On the other hand, if you are sensitive to loss in your own life, you may swing too far in the opposite direction and push the family to resolve these issues, in part, at least, because of your own needs. Supervision in these cases can be helpful in sorting out the personal from the clinical.

The simple, honest approach, of course, is to talk about loss directly. To ask the family what they sense they're losing or fear they may lose puts the topic on the table and helps them to see that moving forward always involves leaving something else behind. This kind of talk not only keeps the family, as well as yourself, from being discouraged by the sudden stall in progress, but opens the door to the larger subject of grief within the family's experience. You can explore past losses and successful transitions. As these old emotions are stirred, rise to the surface, and are finally expressed, these past losses begin to heal and the family's emotional range has another opportunity to grow.

• *Take a break.* As the family improves, they can get burned out on the routine of treatment itself. Just as taking planned rests from intensive physical exercise allows muscles to recover and hence grow, taking a break or reducing sessions in therapy can allow the family to integrate what they have learned, practice skills on their own away from your watchful eye, and increase their own psychological muscles.

If Teresa is pretty much holding her own, having her check in with you every other week or so may be fine. If the family seems to have reached a satisfactory plateau, consider and discuss with them your moving toward some form of case management with the option to return for more intensive work as the need arises. Rather than viewing this as abandonment, families often see this as a graduation of sorts, an endorsement of their growing capability. It also gives you an opportunity to see just how much support they really need.

• *Be brave.* Courage remains the most basic antidote to all this stuckness and backsliding—staying close to the family's and your own anxiety even as distractions arise or new skills gradually take hold, being honest and clear when ambivalence and grief begin to seep out beneath the behavioral changes, challenging both the family and yourself to resist the temptations of lapsing back into the old familiar patterns. By your willingness to continue to move ahead the family is able to do the same.

Keep in mind, however, that courage itself doesn't change the basic landscape. The plodding through new problems, the reassessment, reclassification, and reeducation will remain part of this middle stage. The going, in spite of your best efforts, may at times seem slow and stretch on longer than you at first thought.

HIDDEN SABOTAGE

What makes the family's slipping, sliding, and backtracking manageable is your ability as an outsider to the system to see the process unfold. The greater danger of the middle stage occurs when these same dynamics go underground—when you and family become emotionally intertwined and become part of the system, or when you put up your own roadblocks to just how far the family can go. Here are some of the dangers to avoid:

- *Induction into the system.* In the room with you are Bill and Helen and their three children. The presenting problem is eight-year-old Joey's tendency to play with matches (he was caught trying to light the living room curtains on fire one day), but this is just the latest of many crisis that keep the family in turmoil. You've already decided that Bill needs to take a more active role in parenting, that Helen is overwhelmed and depressed, that communication between the parents is lousy, that ten-year-old Patricia is parentified and barely keeping her head above water, and that four-year-old Tom is likely to follow in his brother's path. You've decided that your initial goals are to pull Bill back into the family process, open and clarify communication, and begin a problem-solving process among everyone.

But as soon as you ask how their week was, a verbal free-for-all erupts. All of the kids at the same time start telling their version of the story of how a hole got knocked in the wall of the kids' room. Helen chimes in and says that she suspects that Joey did it on purpose; Bill tries to pipe in but is quickly drowned out. You play referee and try to have everyone take a turn without interruption by the others; you try to separate and make sense of the stories, but before this incident is resolved, Helen is off on another, with the kids following verbally right behind. The best you can muster is keep everyone from talking at once.

This kind of immersion into the family process, of becoming swept up and away, is fairly common, especially among beginning therapists. Rather than leading the process, you, the clinician, are limping behind, caught in the swirl of family interactions. Whether it is due to your lack of skills, timidity, or both, the problem at home is replayed over and over again there in your office. The family does more of the same, while you are left feeling overrun, overwhelmed, confused. Eventually you wind up feeling just as impotent to change things as they do.

Sometimes, however, rather than becoming emotionally washed away, you step up and end up stepping into one of the family roles. You may, for example, join with Helen and actually stand in for the inactive Bill by scolding Joey, backing up Helen's rules, putting the lid on Tom. Or you may identify with one of the children, and find yourself encouraging Joey to vent his anger right there and then in the room. If there has been a family loss recently—the death of grandparent, a divorce and the leaving of the father—you may, with the family's silent blessing, fill those empty shoes. Once locked into the role, you no longer have to struggle as an outsider, and the family no longer has to figure out what to do with you. Seat down in that empty chair, grab a plate, have some dinner, join in. The old process remains the same; only the face has changed.

This filling of the void is a lure on both sides that, like triangulation, makes for a quick and easy reduction of anxiety all around. From among the choices that the family offers, it's usually easy to find a role that fits your psychological make-up. Even though you think you're working, not much work is really going on. Even though the family knows they're in therapy, it all feels strangely familiar. You're no longer pulling against the family's grain and the family is no longer threatened by questions or comments that make them feel uncomfortable.

This kind of unconscious seduction is, of course, very different from the conscious, deliberate taking of sides—for example, specifically backing up Helen as a way of modeling such behavior for Bill, or giving words to the anger that you suspect Patricia may be feeling but is not saying. In situations like this you are flexible, rather than entrenched; you're clear with the family and yourself as to the what and why of your actions; you're able and ready to pull back or move to another role as the need arises.

• *Parallel process.* Helen yells at Joey, Joey fights with Tom, Tom kicks the dog. The dog bites Tom, Tom hits Joey, Joey steals Patricia's hairbrush, Patricia runs to Mom. Off to counseling steps Mom, who now turns to you, the clinician. The emotional buck gets passed up and down the line, as the patterns of action and reaction are played out over and over again. Just as it is easy for you to get caught up in the swirl of emotions and roles, it's easy to step into line and pass the buck yourself, to your supervisor, rather than stopping it. As soon as the session is over, you're in her office talking about your experience with the family, and sounding just as much in crisis and overwhelmed as they do.

What the good supervisor does at this point is recognize what is happening, do the stopping, and push the process back down the line. She does this by treating the overwhelmed clinician the same way he or she needs to respond to the overwhelmed family. She helps the clinician see the parallels, and empowers the clinician to do the same with the parent.

But, unfortunately, the wave cannot only roll up from the family, but also roll over them from above. If that same supervisor is under a lot of pressure by the agency head to shorten waiting lists or increase revenues, or if the clinician, new to the job, is under probation and feels enormous performance pressure from the supervisor, it doesn't take much for all this anxiety to work its way down and get dumped on the family. Rather than the clinician remaining cool and collected, the clinician is breathing down the parents' necks, pressuring them to shape up and get their act together or pay their bill on time, displacing on them everything he or she feels. Because of the power of the clinician as a role model, it's easy then for the parents to pass this same anxiety down to the children, who then may take it out on each other, the dog, the cat, or the kids sitting next to them in class.

Needless to say, all this can easily get the family off track and worsen their woes. Rather than therapy being a safe place to try new behaviors, it becomes instead a forum for the clinician's or agency's own emotional chaos. Making it all the worse is the clinician's inability to see the impact he or she is having. Few families have the courage or skill to tell the clinician to keep his or her projections to him- or herself, or the self-confidence to really believe that what's happening isn't their fault. If not corrected by the clinician, they'll eventually drop out, convinced once and for all that they are hopeless or that therapy isn't worth a damn.

• *Countertransference.* Both induction and parallel process reflect countertransference issues in that the clinician is ensnared by a family's particular dynamics and pulled into the family system without his or her awareness. But there is another, more generalized form of counter-transference that takes the form of blind spots and roadblocks which serve to emotionally protect the clinician, but limit the family's therapeutic progress.

You may, for example, be easily intimidated by men such as Bill who have high-power jobs, are older than you, or seem controlling. Rather than dealing up front with your own anxiety, you may find rationalizations to exclude him from the therapy: "It's too bad that he has to work so late, but rather than cancel, the rest of us can go ahead and meet without him." If he is there in the room, you may simply ignore him (thereby also replicating the family process and providing a double whammy), join with Helen and gang up against him, use her to express your own anger or fear vicariously, or silence Helen and act ingratiating toward him as a way of winning his favor.

Similarly, you may have difficulty dealing with problems of sexual or verbal abuse or depression, stemming not from lack of skill, but from deeper personal reactions; rather than confronting these topics and your emotions, the topic is never raised or is minimized, even when it's clear to an outsider it's important. Perhaps your supervisor notices a pattern across your caseload, or you may vaguely sense yourself when you look back on your work that you tend to only go so far in the course of therapy. With the help of innumerable rationalizations (the mother needs to see someone individually, the family isn't ready to deal with Dad's addiction, they aren't working, they need time to consolidate the gains that they have made), relationships are cut off just when the client becomes too dependent, too provocative, too angry, too something—which triggers your own anxiety and personal emotional bottom line. Rather than pressing forward, you, in self-defense, quit.

All this can be subtle and difficult to untangle because it is below conscious awareness and potentially filled with anxiety. It's this anxiety, not lack of skill, and the anxiety-binding behaviors it generates that are the drivers here for such widespread, across-the-board patterns of avoidance, under- or overreaction, or vicarious expression of emotion by others. The anxiety distorts what the clinician sees and hears, and turns a rationale into a rationalization that limits or undermines the family's progress.

• *Collusion.* Finally, there is a form of sabotage that arises not out of your immersion or filling in of already established roles, but from the therapy culture that you and the family together create. Basically, you all fall into a rut. Each session, for example, follows the same format, propelled by the same questions or comments—"How was your week?"; "Let's pick up off where we left off last time." Then Dad complains, Mom discounts him, you mediate and give generally the same advice, which is never fully followed. Or the mother comes in complaining about one of the children, but this is only a learned warm-up to her talking about her ex-husband, or for you simply to ask questions about her past. The content is less important than the predictable spending of time together or the pseudo-intimacy feelings.

Collusion is in place when the therapy has lost its cutting edge and everyone silently agrees not to change. While there's the appearance of movement, little is actually changing; form has superseded function. Everyone is comfortable rather than challenged. The emotions generated within the session (the mother's feelings of closeness and intimacy, the father's feelings of resentment toward his wife, the clinician's feeling of power or indispensability) become the new comfortable emotions that fuel and maintain the therapy's roles and patterns. The therapy rolls along, sometimes for years; its only value is its stability.

This is not to say that stability can't be legitimate goal, especially for chaotic families. But it's not a legitimate goal when it helps the clinician avoid the confrontation and risk taking the family needs in order to change, when it is supported by rationalizations rather than realistic family needs. Like the other forms of sabotage, collusion is a subtle process that if gone unchecked quickly undermines the therapeutic process.

COUNTERING SABOTAGE

Ideally all of this should never go unchecked, and usually it doesn't. One of the primary lines of defense is good supervision. Because the supervisor is further removed from the family system, he or she is able to see the patterns that the clinician may be blind to, can detect the parallel process rolling his or her way by the clinician's presentation of the case, knows the clinician well enough to recognize when distorted reactions are once again surfacing.

Even if the supervisor doesn't have it all worked out but suspects that the clinician is more entangled than he or she intended or is rationalizing his or her behavior, by simply raising the issue ("I wonder if you are stepping in for this mother who is so passive"; "I wonder if the way you feel now as you are talking is very much the way the father felt"; "I notice you have a hard time dealing with adolescents who act like this"), the statement or question itself becomes a crowbar for prying up what is embedded below the surface. What was hidden is now out in the open; the unconscious is made conscious and loses its power.

As the clinician, you can also do your own prying. By knowing yourself and the individual family you can anticipate the holes, traps, and roles that can ensnare you. By being familiar with your own weaknesses, you can stay alert to the cutoffs, avoidances, and attractions; the overresponsibility; your need for clients to express what you cannot. By being sensitive to the larger patterns of your work, you will be able to recognize and emotionally separate the rationale from the rationalization. You'll be able to tell whose needs you are most trying to meet.

Finally, you can solicit the family's help with this process as well. By making the time to reevaluate the therapeutic contract at regular intervals, they (and you) can have the opportunity to say aloud whether everything is on course. If there has been an imbalance in the family sessions, if one member has been ignored or felt ganged up on, or if new goals need to be set, here is the chance for it to all get out in the open, rather than the family dealing with their confusion or resentment by dropping out or become passive. During these discussions you need to be sensitive to the nonverbal as well as verbal communication of everyone in the room. If you are only willing to hear what you want to hear, what you'll get is exactly what you want, unfortunately, at cost to the family.

But the simple solution is always the most reliable. If sabotage is driven by the avoidance of anxiety, it is the presence of anxiety, your ability to stay at the edge of change—in the process, in the room, in your self—that is the best antidote. When the process is gets too easy, too comfortable, or too predicable for too long, this should raise the alarm that something may be going offtrack, that the family's needs may be compromised, that you have lost your power as an outside agent to affect change. Even if you're not sure at that moment what the right thing to do is, return to the basics of honesty and courage. Slow down, define, take responsibility for yourself. This will help you recenter yourself and the process on the right path, and lead you and the family to where you need to be.

FIRST AID FOR THE AWFUL SESSION

No matter how good a job you do at confronting the patterns of sabotage, induction, and collusion, at some point you are bound to have one of those absolutely awful sessions that every therapist has. These have less to do with the family's or your own dynamics and more to do with the simple fact that you're having a bad day: You were awake most of the night before because your kid threw up every 15 minutes, perhaps you had a blowout with your spouse just as you were walking out the door about the dog peeing on the carpet *again*, or your mother called last night to say that, oh, by the way, she felt a lump in her breast, and though it's probably nothing, she's scheduling a doctor's appointment for first thing in the morning, but don't you worry about it.

So you walk into work feeling groggy, irritable, or worried, and actually the last thing you want to do is to listen to more people and their problems. But you do, and then Henry makes that same smirk he always does when his wife Betty talks about the trouble Freddie gave her that week, and you feel like clobbering the guy. Of course you don't, but you do come down on him pretty hard, and naturally, all he does is glare at you while denying feeling anything, leaving you feeling even more frustrated. Or Denise starts with her whiny pleas to the boys to stop arguing, but you're so tired that you just let it go until before you know it the boys are running out the door and down the hallway. She falls apart and starts crying, but you can't help her because you're off down the hall trying to find out which direction the kids went.

These kind of sessions can be hard to shake off. They leave you feeling angry and guilty and worried. You kick yourself for being so mean or lazy, for getting into this stupid kind of work, for getting a dog, for getting married, for that matter. You're mad at this family for doing the same thing over and over again in spite of your best efforts for the last six sessions to try and get them to do something different. You're worried they'll never come back, and hope to God they never do.

Slow down. It's not the end of the world. First of all, give yourself a break. Sure, you could have done a better job, but you did the best you could at the time. Mistakes are called mistakes rather than tragedies because you can correct them. Take a couple a deep breaths and figure out what you need to do next.

Did the session leave you so concerned about the impact on the family that you need to do something before the next appointment? Is Henry apt to be steaming mad and take it out on Betty or the kids all week? Will he decide not to come back? Is Denise feeling so wrecked that she's likely to collapse all together and lose all the ground she's made? Will she get depressed and start having suicidal thoughts again?

If you feel that someone in the family will act out or emotionally go into a tailspin, think he or she might but aren't sure, or just feel uncomfortable about it all, do something. Call up the family later in the day to see how they're doing, find out what they're thinking, apologize to Henry, reassure Denise. You don't need to spend an hour on the phone—you can talk more about what happened at the next session—but do some crisis intervention. If you can't reach them, leave a message on the answering machine asking them to call you, or simply saying that you realize that it was a tough session, you're sorry, and you're just checking in, or write them a brief note and mail it. Sound concerned, not angry, say what you think they may be thinking or feeling, but don't obsess or feel helpless. Do something.

If you feel that yes, they'll be back, and it's not urgent to talk to them, wait till the next session. Start the session cleaning up the last one: "Before we get started on whatever you wanted to cover, I'd like to talk a bit about what happened last week." Then talk—apologize if you feel an apology is in order, talk about your feelings in the process ("I felt frustrated when . . . "), talk about yourself ("I realize I didn't say much last week; I was preoccupied because . . . "). Then ask the family to give their impressions of the session: Denise says she felt overwhelmed; Henry didn't understand why you kept asking the same thing over and over again, and frankly it was bugging the hell out of him. Or, often following the family's established pattern, they may say nothing: "I just felt a bit overwhelmed, again," says Denise, "but I was okay." "No," says Henry, "I don't remember anything being wrong." Only later, after their trust and assertiveness increase, may they say something about it.

Regardless of what they do or don't say, you're modeling something important—how to admit and repair mistakes, how to take responsibility, how to communicate clearly when communication has broken down, how to repair relationships. This can be a powerful experience for families who always sweep things under the rug, never apologize or always blame, or never talk about talking. Once again you're approaching anxiety, you're dealing with the therapeutic derailment by looking at it squarely with honesty, clarity, and empathy. It's the most and the best you can do.

With all the movement in the therapy practice brought on by managed care and the press of brief work in recent years, the traditional image of the middle stage seems to be changing; it is less the long, flat stretch that it used to be and more a way station between the beginning and termination. But even if the stages of therapy are more compressed, the challenge to appreciate the integrity of each stage remains.

To say to yourself or to a family that we have reached the middle of the therapy, that this is a plateau and not the end, that repetition and relearning are the nature of this time is to define and map the contours of the change process itself. It's shaped by your theory and at a deeper level by your own values and beliefs about your role, the purpose of therapy, and the developmental process. How you think about the flow of the therapy process, in this stage and the others, will affect what you, and the family, will come to expect and eventually discover.

Looking Within: Chapter 7 Exercises

Just as the exercises of the last chapter focused on skills and issues related to the beginning stage of treatment, these exercises focus on those of the middle stage. Once again take the risk and give them a try.

1. Think about a couple of ongoing or past cases. How do you decide when to stop with a case, when to stick with it? How much do you believe change is occurring even when it is not evident? How do you know when you are taking too much responsibility for change within the family?

2. Countertransference. Think again about the kind of clients are most difficult for you to work with. How do you respond to these clients? What role do you usually take? How does this role limit your therapeutic flexibility? Does it offer any therapeutic advantages? How could your supervisor or therapist best help you understand and broaden your options?

3. What kind of problems are emotionally the most difficult for you? How do you respond to them? What is your emotional bottom line? What kind of rationalizations are you susceptible to? How do handle loss, in yourself, in others? Again, are these indicators of unresolved issues from your past that need your attention? Who do you feel comfortable talking to about them?

4. Increase your awareness of parallel process by noticing it in settings outside of clinical work. Notice in a store, for example, how a child will complain to the mother, and the mother will then turn and complain to the father, or at work the way the director's urgency over some matter will trickle down through the supervisor to the staff, or even at home when your spouse lectures or your child whines to you and you pass it along and do the same to someone else. Practice stopping the process.

[8]

Endings

ENOUGH ALREADY?

Endings, in therapy, in life, are a culmination of the process and products of all that has gone on before. Like the beginning and middle stages of treatment, they reflect your own theory, values, and personality, as well as your patterns, but, more than that, they reflect the two-way street between client and clinician that is the therapeutic process. Good endings, just like good beginnings and middles, require that special kind of clinical sensitivity to yourself and the family's needs and patterns.

So where and when do you draw the line? When is enough, enough? When they stop bringing in problems? When the I.P. is no longer the I.P.? But what about the trouble the couple continues to have if they try to talk to each other for more than five minutes? What about the mother's occasional claim that the father drinks too much? Should you try and tackle that, even though everything else seems to be going along okay? And what about the growing dependency that you sense the family has on you? How do you get them to see that they can really manage things on their own without your cutting things off and having them fall back to zero in a week?

I know what you are thinking. In all too many cases you never really get a chance to ask yourself these questions. Half the families, it seems, never make it beyond three sessions. They decide the fee is too high, or find that the insurance won't cover your treatment after all, or that managed care has a five-session cap. Or the only one who ever makes it in is the mother, and after a few weeks of this, she decides that she isn't going to give a damn if no one else in the family does. Or to everyone's surprise Sally's dad decided that she could come out and spend the whole summer with him three states away in Iowa, and she left town last Friday, so we guess there's nothing really to work on. Or after two sessions everyone in the family decides they're better—Bobby did get up and get himself to school last Monday and only had one fight (which he didn't start!), and, besides, dad's going to be out of town for three weeks because of work, and we'll give you a call when he gets back. The family has quit after going less than a quarter lap around the therapy track.

But sometimes it's not that way. There are times when endings do come in a planned way, when the word termination is actually spoken aloud and discussed, when the good ending not only brings a psychological closure to a good therapy, but completes a healing deep within. Even if the formal endings rarely come with the hug or pat on the shoulder in the doorway or the long slow walk down the office corridor for the last time, endings really are important enough that they should be part of your beginning, part of your assessment, part of your vision, and, you hope, part of the family's vision as well.

Endings should be anticipated; they rarely should be a surprise to you. Just as your own theory tells you about the beginning and middle stages, it becomes the starting point for defining the endings as well. If you are doing brief therapy, or have a 10-session cap on treatment, the ending will be fairly clear. If you see your role as lifelong consultant—giving families a boost up to get over the latest developmental hurdle, then pulling back and waiting in the wings until the next cycle arises—you can share this vision with the family from the onset and map a course together. If you view therapy as a process of peeling away layers, going ever deeper into the family or individual's psyche, then what others call an ending may be for you only a plateau of the middle. Your theory, whatever it may be, establishes the parameters of the work.

Endings should not be a surprise to the family either. The expected time of treatment should all be out in the open, all part of the therapeutic contract. If you work under a session limit because of your or the agency's approach, let the family know at the first session so they can narrow their focus and understand what is expected. If you only do long-term work (for example, a year or more), be up front about this and help them understand your reasons (e.g., your belief in the need to resolve underlying past issues). This will help the family appreciate your process, pace, and focus, or decide that this isn't what they want at all and keep you both from becoming frustrated.

If your work is somewhere in the middle, varying from a few sessions to a few months, depending upon the nature of the problem and the family, say that, or simply tell the family how often the contract will be reviewed (for example, taking a few minutes every five sessions or so to see if everything is on target). However you decide to handle the therapeutic time frame, let the family know what it is.

Your assessment of the family should include an assessment of their endings. If the family seems to be one that lives from crisis to the next, it's a good bet that they'll be ready to leave once the current crisis is over. If they report dropping out of past therapy when the therapist starting asking questions about the marriage, which had nothing to do, they felt, with their son's problems, you can suspect that the marriage again could be the hot-button issue that gets them out the door. If the family describes a pattern of avoiding grief or intimacy by finding reasons to get angry and prematurely breaking off relationships, you can anticipate this shift with you and be prepared to try and cut them off at the pass.

Don't keep your thoughts to yourself. It's valuable to talk to the family about termination as part and parcel of their other family patterns. If the Wilson parents, for example, describe a pattern of cutting off relationships when they don't get their way (pulling their child out of private school when their son isn't given the classes they think he should have, not talking to relatives who don't take their side in a dispute over an inheritance), you may want to wonder aloud whether they might find themselves wanting to drop out of therapy if at some point you too don't seem be going along with what they expect. Similarly, in the Taylor family, the father describes his tendency to pull away from everyone and hole up in his workshop whenever conflict arises at home. Highlighting this pattern and expressing your fear that he will stop coming to therapy if the sessions seem too volatile makes his cutoff more transparent and less likely to happen.

By helping the family to recognize their ways of using endings to cope with difficult situations and emotions, their behavior loses some of its seductive and automatic quality. By discussing their pattern of termination well in advance, you are posing to them a possible new option, and your confrontation about the process seems less of a personal attack. As in other areas of their lives, you are inviting them to see and stop their own pattern; you are challenging them to go against their own grain in order to increase their ways of coping with and creating relationships.

All this mapping of time frames and patterns isn't any guarantee, of course, that it all will turn out the way you think it should. With some families there seems to be a running struggle over when and who pulls the plug. Even though Mary, for example, might no longer be hanging out with that 20-year-old biker, you think it would be good for the parents to iron out some unresolved divorce issues if they are to keep the same problems from coming up with the younger children; they, however, are ready to quit. Even though Sam and Helen are talking and making decisions better, Sam's underlying depression, you feel, still keeps the relationship from becoming more intimate, yet both of them feel that all is fine.

How much of this is client reluctance to engage in further treatment, therapist reluctance to end, or a power struggle over who runs the show depends again upon your theory, your view of the problem, and the scope of therapy. Your task, and the limits of your power, lie in making the family aware of your perspective, the clinical options you see, the rationale, and the possible consequences of each of them. The contract, in order to remain viable, continually needs to be clarified and renegotiated, with the endpoints clear.

Then there are the ethical issues. While you can't force people to continue when they don't want to, on the other side, you can't abandon them if they are unstable and clinically still need your help. The most common situation, perhaps, is a clinician's move to end treatment because the client's insurance has suddenly ended or capped out, and contracts with the insurance company forbid the clinician from negotiating a lower fee. But the same problem arises should the clinician decide that he or she is not the best suited in skill or style to provide the services the client needs. If the client is in crisis—the dad is suicidal, the daughter is beginning to decompensate—the clinician is ethically responsible to maintain services until an appropriate transfer to another clinician can be arranged. Leaving a psychologically vulnerable client high and dry is against the ethical standards of the various therapy professions. When in doubt, talk it over with a supervisor or respected colleague.

QUITTING TIME

No matter how and where you envision the end, there are plenty of signs to tell you when a family is ready to quit. One of the best, of course, is that everything is better. The presenting problem is resolved, as are the underlying factors responsible for its creation. You'll notice a relaxation, even boredom in the sessions—the edgy overreaction and crisis mentality have dissipated. Conversations fall to small talk, clients start forgetting some of their appointments or find reasons to spread them out, and you find yourself wondering what you should do next. The sense of purpose and direction seem unclear.

What you do with this is say what you have been thinking and feeling—that things are better and have been steady for awhile, that you're wondering what they want to do. Generally at this point the family members start nodding their heads and give a sigh of relief because they finally have permission to say what they have been also thinking for the past month. Once you broach the subject of termination they're ready to make a beeline for the door.

If, however, you put this discussion off too long, some families will just drop out. Even though they're doing better, they may not have the courage to tell you they want to leave: They may be worried about how you would react, they have too many mixed feelings about it themselves. Rather than approach this anxiety, it's easier for them simply to stop coming.

This awkward, unsettled ending can dissuade some families from calling you in the future, even if they would like to return, and the longer the time the greater the awkwardness and anxiety. Three years later you'll meet them in the checkout line at the supermarket, and if they don't look away or head for a different aisle, they'll casually mention how well everyone is doing. To finish this unfinished business and give them permission to come back, it's a good idea to always do some form of follow-up.

Obviously, not all families leave because they're all better. Some are a little better and that is enough for them, or not much better at all, but problems on the job, financial pressures, or illness take over and push therapy to the bottom of their to-do list. Again, while dropping therapy can often can be seen as another example of a family's crisis mentality and difficulty with setting priorities, it also can be a realistic response to the events in their life. The loss of a job, a serious illness, the sudden death of a parent—all life transitions that may possibly benefit from the therapy support—can be so overwhelming and emotionally demanding that they monopolize the family's energy and resources. Therapy, rather than being a source of support, feels like another obligation to worry about, at a time when additional worries are the last things they need. While some families will make the effort to describe all this to you in a last session, a majority of others will not. Instead they will fail to show up at or cancel a series of appointments, or leave several garbled messages with the receptionist, saying they will call back when they can. Again, a follow-up from you will encourage them to return when they are ready.

Finally, there are those who are ready to end because things, as they see it, aren't better, or may be even worse than when they first started— Vinny was having some trouble going to school, but now Andrea is talking about how depressed she is and the parents are fighting like never before. They may blame you for stirring up trouble, or feel invaded by your seemingly constant prodding. Or they have already spent $500 and you're still asking questions, not giving them enough advice, or making anything better. A few might be angry enough to tell you how they feel, but most will just call up and cancel because of car trouble. They never call back.

Sometimes you have to agree with them. The therapy actually hasn't been going well. You were hoping things would get rolling in that next session when Grandma and Grandpa were scheduled to show up and talk about their own marital woes, or after you got the results of the psychological testing on Vinny. Other times the problem is one of expectations or timing. Somehow their vision of the process and your own were never clarified or reconciled. They expected you to see Vinny by himself and fix him in two sessions, and here you are bringing in everybody and asking a lot of stupid questions about their childhoods or how they feel after a fight. Or perhaps you spent three sessions doing an assessment, and in the fourth you're turning up the heat on Mom and pushing her to make decisions that she has never had to struggle with before. Their anxiety goes through the roof, they don't understand the rationale for it all, and they decide to leave their trauma making to home.

It's hard not to feel angry with yourself if a family pulls out after a bad session; it's even harder when you thought things were going fine. The therapy may have been more important to you than to them, or in spite of gains they still felt that they weren't getting what they wanted. Feeling rejected as a clinician is no small thing, especially if your self-confidence is shaky or if a lot of your own identity is caught up in your work and how well you do it.

It's unrealistic to expect there always to be a perfect balance in the therapeutic relationship. You're a person first, therapist second, and there are always some families that you like more than others, some you may like more than they like you. If they suddenly leave, it's easy for all those little kid feelings of being bad, wanting a second chance, making things right to be stirred up within you. You have the urge to call them up, see what's wrong, have a chance to explain what you did and what you meant, to encourage them to come back.

At first glance such thoughts and fantasies may not seem to you like bad ideas, and on some level they may not be, but realize as well that they are being amplified by your own countertransference feelings of loss. Go talk to your supervisor first to help you sort out your sense of rejection and loss from the family's real clinical needs. If this seems to be happening frequently, if your commitment to the family always seems to be greater than theirs, this is a sign that some old issue for you is being stirred up. It's probably compromising your ability to do your work effectively; it's time to consider some therapy for yourself.

How you actually decide to follow up when they drop out depends on your own individual style and relationship with the family. Some therapists like to call and some families don't mind this at all; the connection by human voice, the ability to talk and listen becomes not only a good way of reaching out to the family, but possibly of reaching a more personal closure. Other families feel this is invasive. Your calling feels like you're checking up on them, tracking them down, putting them on the spot. It only encourages them to make up all kinds of transparent excuses and promises that they'll come in next time. Leaving a planned phone message (e.g., calling their home when you know they are at work), provides the intimacy of your voice without the putting them on the spot.

Others like to send a follow-up note. While writing lacks the intimacy of voice contact, the client can read the letter at his or her leisure, or reread it if anything is unclear. The note can be simple and matter of fact ("Sorry you couldn't make our last appointment, give me a call so we can schedule another") or more descriptive and therapeutic ("I've wondered if you feel that the therapy hasn't been helping as much as you hoped it would. Perhaps it would be worthwhile for us to talk about this, to help me understand better what you're needing, and what I could do differently"). If you feel the family has stopped because they have quit for now, you can say that since you haven't heard from them that you're assuming things are fine, but they are welcome to give you a call should something come up in the future.

Like other actions you take with a family, your response is never neutral. Whatever approach you choose and follow-up decision you make, it should be driven by clinical concerns and knowledge of the family, rather than your own awkwardness or convenience. You are still serving as a model of good communication. It's important to say as clearly and as sensitively as possible what you think the client might be feeling and thinking as well as what you would like to do. In effect, you are providing in written or verbal form your half of the dialogue that would ideally happen if the client came in to the office. Give the client a few weeks to respond. If you haven't heard, follow up with whatever you normal procedure is, for example, simply close the case and document your actions in their chart, send a letter telling the family that you are closing their case.

CLOSING YOUR DOOR

Of course there are times when you're the one who wants to terminate. You feel like they're not getting anywhere or your supervisor tells you the waiting list is three miles long and you need to make room for the new clients. Perhaps they never really follow through with your suggestions, or the people have rubbed you the wrong way since you first met them in the waiting room, or you feel that they are setting you up to testify in an ugly court battle. Or maybe it's a matter of skill, or lack of it: After a few sessions you realize that the problem is more complex than you thought— the 14-year-old is bulimic or the mother shows signs of multiple personality.

And so you literally jump for joy or sigh with relief when it snows or they call up to cancel because of the flu. You put off returning their phone calls, or call back, let the phone the ring once and hang up. You find yourself sending follow-up letters with the wrong zip code, or you seem a little bit too enthusiastic when they suggest having the school psychologist work with Susie at school instead of spending the money to see you. Short of paying them not to come back, or quitting your job and leaving town, you'll do just about anything not have to go on.

Or perhaps it's less about your skill and more about reevaluating the family's needs. The father needs inpatient drug treatment before any progress can be made in family therapy; the mother needs social services in order to get environmentally stable before any therapy can be effective; the son is becoming psychotic and needs hospitalization for evaluation, medication, and stabilization; the family is too chaotic to effectively use or even get into outpatient services—home-based services would better fit their needs. Your role changes from a family therapist to a referral source.

Whatever the reason for the change, it's time for some supervisory consultation. If the family needs a shift in services for clinical reasons, your supervisor needs to be aware of your thinking and plan. If the urge to escape from certain of your clients is part of a larger pattern for you, you may decide you need to work it out in your own therapy while you continue to see the family. If you lack particular skills, you may decide that with enough supervisory support and skill coaching, you can work through it with them. If you and supervisor agree that your reactions are interfering with your ability to work with them, or that you are clinically over your head, you may need to pull out.

Of course, there will usually come the day when you really do need to leave, not just the family but the work—you've been fired (no, not really); you're going back to school to study 13th-century English literature or septic tank repair; or you're getting married and moving to Oklahoma. These are easier to explain to the family in some ways, but often only a bit less so. Many families already have old issues around abandonment, and your leaving only stirs them up. You need to give the family as much notice as possible, you need to help the family members sort through these feelings, you need to give them permission to get angry at you for pulling out (i.e., ask, "Are you angry about my leaving?") or angry at you for having the flexibility to do with your life what they feel they cannot. When handled well, these kinds of leavings can be invaluable experiences for mending old wounds.

Honesty rules once again. While it's tempting to attempt to drive those difficult families away with your neglect, or, worse perhaps, your rationalization that they really don't need to come any more, it's dishonest and destructive. Instead you need to use all your good communication skills (the "I" statements; talking about yourself, not them; talking about feelings, as well as facts). Take responsibility for the reasons that have to do with you, say why other services or another therapist would serve them better, honestly tell them how you see the situation. Then listen. Make sure that they don't blame themselves or misunderstand and think that they need to try harder, and offer to talk some more about it if necessary. Give them options for transferring if they want to continue and have a plan to make it happen; don't abandon them, especially if they are in crisis, until something else is in place.

Consider easing the transition to another therapist, to a hospital, by personally going with them the first time. This gives you a chance to describe in front of the family member your summary of the work and the problem, or gives the client the opportunity to sort through his or her feelings and describe your relationship and work together to the new clinician. This not only provides some closure, but helps the new person be aware of and sensitive to the loss issues that may arise as he or she begins. The more the family has invested in the process and the relationship, the more important all this is.

GOOD ENDINGS

Regardless of the circumstances surrounding any case, what you are always ideally shooting for are good terminations. They are like any other good death—they leave enough time and space around them for everything that needs to get done and said, actually to get done and said. The basic elements include everything you've read about in all those textbooks— give the family notice; set an ending date; explore the feelings about the leaving; expect testing, crises, and everything seeming to fall apart; better yet, predict the crises for them so they realize that it is all part of the ending process; review all the skills learned and progress made. Help the family see that their own feelings of loss and abandonment don't take away from their ability to go it on their own.

Most clinicians use one of two basic ending formats. One is the decisive "do it and leave" approach—set an ending date several weeks or months in the future, meet at the same regular pace (weekly, biweekly) and stick with the plan no matter what. The date is negotiated with the family and may be built around another convenient marker—summer vacations, start of the school year, and the like. The other approach is the "fade away"—spacing out sessions over increasingly longer periods of time, for example, weekly, then monthly for a couple of months, then again in three months, then in six months if it is needed.

What you choose depends upon your own preference and the needs of the family. The "do it and leave" has a counting-down effect that's clear and definitive for the family, but can raise anxiety, which in turn can promote crises as the count gets shorter—that's not a reason not to do it, but a reason to be prepared. The "fade away" reduces some of the anxiety by giving the family an opportunity to see for themselves that they can really handle things on their own. But it also can give the impression that the ending is less defined, more open-ended; in their anxiety it's easy to go into denial and pretend that it's never going to happen. Potentially you could wind up stretching things out so long that other developmental life events pop up (Would you believe it, Jane just got pregnant!), fueling the need to continue monitoring or to crank up treatment up. You can make this the last final challenge for the family and suggest the format that moves against their grain and encourages them to incorporate the skills they have learned. Oftentimes you can simply give the family a choice of formats, and the clinician needs only to enforce it.

Of course, enforcement can sometimes seem difficult when the termination crises start to mount. The best approach is one that is matter-of-fact: Reassure the family that they know what to do; coach them through problem-solving the situation, intervening in as minimal a way as possible; and predict and interpreting the crisis in light of the upcoming termination. Generally, if things are handled in this way the first couple of times, the crises will rapidly diminish.

This doesn't mean that you may not have doubts—maybe they need more time, more support, maybe I'm throwing them out the door and they're not ready. Maybe you're right. There are some families—those with severe environmental hardships, parents with lower intelligence, for example—that may struggle with the application of skills without some ongoing support. This becomes a clinical decision. You may want to do check-ins via phone or in person on a regular basis, or refer the family for ongoing case management. But it's also possible that your reservations about termination come more from you—your own separation anxiety, your own loss, your own sense of inflated importance. Talk it over with your supervisor or a colleague whose opinion you trust. Take the time the separate out your reactions from theirs.

It's often good to have some form of a closing ritual. This is especially true for families with whom you have worked intensely—home-based cases, cases you've seen for a long period of time—or where there are young children who are not fully understanding the ending process. Drawing a picture all together, doing a formalized recitation of the changes each has made, sharing a meal (this is easy and usually quite appropriate with home-based work), doing a closing experiential exercise (a guided fantasy about the future or about giving each other symbolic gifts) all have a way of bringing together and acknowledging the mixture of emotions that endings bring.

It's always useful to have some kind of joint review of what the clients have learned. This allows both you and them actually to articulate the progress made and, more importantly, helps them recognize the skills learned. These skills are what they can draw on when similar problems arise in the future; you can underscore them in the discussion.[1]

As you have done all along, you once again set the pace, model the way to do it. You're the one who needs to talk about the mixed feelings that both you and they have. You're the one who keeps everyone and everything on task so that distractions don't derail this part of the process any more than any of the others. You're the one who with honesty and caring shows the family how people can leave and continue with their lives.

The door is always left open, for another round of work, for problem solving, for a quick consultation as the family moves through new stages of development and old issues once again raise their head. Some families, of course, never return. Others make the out-of-the-blue phone call on some Thursday afternoon asking the out-of-the-blue question, sometimes seeking useful information, sometimes just seeing if you're still there. Some come back a year or two or five later for a few sessions or a few months. And once again you start, hoping to pick up where you both left off, but, not surprisingly, finding out that you both have changed. A new beginning with new expectations.

Again the reality of practice makes these good endings rarer than they should be, but when they come they are invaluable for what they offer—the sense of groundedness, completion, and definitiveness. At that last session there's that wonderful sigh and sense that something important here has happened.

---

[1]Another way of approaching this kind of summary is to ask the family to say what they hypothetically could do if they wanted to return things to the way they were before they started treatment.

We have finished our trilogy of the beginning, middle, and end, ideally covering all the basic parameters of family therapy practice. We're now ready to look at the family therapy with specific cases over the course of the developmental cycle.

Looking Within: Chapter 8 Exercises

1. Take a few moments and think back over endings in your own life, those clearly marked—the graduation from high or college, your marriage or divorce, the death of a parent—or those numerous unmarked ones—the way you and your childhood best friend just drifted away, the gradual ending to your relationship with an old boyfriend or girlfriend, the way your father one day called you up for your advice. Try to remember how you felt, the feelings that led you to the ending, the way you handled those emotions, how free you felt showing them to others, how you behaviorally coped in the days and months that followed. See if any of those patterns affect your expectations of termination with clients, affect your own emotional bottom lines in your work.

2. As you did with middles, take the time to think about your notion of termination, your role, your stopping point according to your theory. Are there times when termination has more met your needs than those of the family? How can you increase your awareness of these countertransference reactions when they come up in your work?

3. How do you personally handle rejection? For what types of families, under what circumstances would their leaving be particularly hurtful to you? Imagine talking to one such family, saying how and why you felt the way you did. What personal issues, if any, does this stir up for you?

4. Take the time to think once again about your own needs from doing family therapy, your own needs issues of loss and separa-

tion that may affect your practice, your own ways of avoiding families you do not like.

5. What kind of cases, problems would you automatically consider transferring out because you feel your skills and knowledge are limited? How could you increase those skills?

6. Develop your own termination rituals that reflect your own personality.

[9]

Billy's Got a Problem
KIDS IN THE FAMILY

Billy sits quietly, scanning the toys on the shelf, his arm tucked under the arm of his grandmother, as she describes why they've come to see you. Although he's seven years old, Billy looks five, he's so short and skinny. His blue eyes are clear and bright, but he avoids eye contact with you. He's seems a little bored.

Billy has been with her now for about two months, says Ms. Williams, and she is having a hard time getting him to mind. She always feels like he's pushing her, and thrusts out her big hand to emphasize how she feels. More often than not he'll throw a fit if he doesn't get his own way and, she admits somewhat sheepishly, she sometimes gives in just to settle him down. But settling down isn't what he does too often; he's always doing something. In fact, the only time he's quiet is when he's sitting in front of the TV or sleeping. He's doing well in school, though. No problems there; he likes it, has friends, and seems smart. The grandmother turns her head and smiles at Billy. She looks exhausted.

The grandmother had already supplied some history when she had called: Billy had come to her following a three month's stay in a foster home. He had been living with his mother and her boyfriend, Tom, and his three-year-old half-brother until the night the boyfriend beat the brother to death. The details are unclear; Billy was in the home at the time, but no one knows just how much he saw. His mother told him that his brother had choked to death on a toy. The boyfriend was arrested and convicted of murder and is now serving 15 years in prison. Although present when it happened, Billy's mother was not charged, but Social Services removed Billy from the home. The mother continues to live in the same town she had been, some 200 miles away, and hasn't seen Billy for five months. Ms. Williams is angry at Billy's mother and his father, her son Edward, for ignoring Billy. She's worried about the effects of the death on him, worried about his reluctance to talk about it.

Living with the grandmother is her husband, Ray, who, like her, is in his late 50s, and is out of town several days a week as a truck driver. Also in the home is her middle son, John, who is in his late 20s; he's recently divorced and the father of a three-year-old son whom he rarely sees. Grandmother's youngest son, Ben, is stationed in Thailand in the Air Force. In addition to caring for all these men she also looks after her own elderly parents and runs errands for them daily. No wonder she looks exhausted.

The start of each new case is like standing at the edge of a dense forest. All we can see before us are the faint markings of paths among the trees. As we take the first steps into the wood, gather our impressions and begin to organize them around the client's personality, priorities, and motivation as well as our theory, personality, and interests, we discover that the forest is actually crisscrossed with numerous paths. While we usually assume that there is only one path that takes us where we want to go, we see that there are, in fact, several possibilities.

Together with the family we make choices, trusting our intuitions, following the most pressing needs, closing off one treatment option, trying another, coming back to the first, trying still a third. While our knowledge and experience can give us some idea of what we may expect, it's only by actually working with the family over time, seeing the consequences of our choices, setting and resetting our priorities based upon environmental and psychological changes that we can actually know how close we are to coming out on the other side.

In this chapter and the next we following the story of Billy as it actually unfolded in the course of his therapy. As we reach decision points along the way we'll stop to consider some of the options that were available. As we do, consider how you might decide to proceed in a similar situation.

Start by taking a couple of minutes to develop your own impressions so far:

- If you were seeing this family, what, according to your own theory, would you want to know?
- What is your tentative hypothesis about the cause of Billy's misbehavior?
- What are Billy's and the family's strengths?
- What parenting skills do the grandparents need to effectively manage him?
- What's missing in the family process?
- Where would you focus first?
- How would you make contact with Billy?
- How do you envision the course of therapy?

Here's my short list of brainstorm ideas:

- *Presenting problem.* Billy's testing limits at home and his grandmother is having difficulty managing his behavior. She's also concerned about Billy's reaction to his loss and trauma.
- *Possible family concerns.* It's unclear why Ms. Williams has difficulty setting limits with Billy: Does she lack the parenting skills, or are her emotions—that is, feelings of anxiety or guilt—interfering with putting those skills into action? What about her high level of stress and possible depression? Can her husband Ray and her son John support her by helping with parenting, becoming more involved with Billy? What about Billy's role in the family structure—is he a scapegoat, a vicarious expression of anger for other members of the family? What is the marital relationship between the grandparents like? How has John coped with his own sense of loss surrounding his divorce and son, and what impact has that had on the family? What role can or should Billy's parents play in his recovery?
- *Possible concerns for Billy.* Obviously, Billy's struggling with grief— the loss of mother, father, brother. He may feel guilty about his brother's death and the boyfriend's imprisonment, or feel responsible for his parent's abandoning of him. He may be suffering not only from posttraumatic stress from brother's death, but other violence toward his mother and him that we, as yet, don't know about. Is he identifying with the aggressive boyfriend or does his behavior reflect a typical testing of limits in a home with new rules and structure? Is he clearly depressed, or does he have attention-deficit/hyperactivity disorder or an attachment disorder?

- *Strengths*. Billy's grandmother clearly cares and seems committed to him. The home environment, although stressful, overall seems stable. Ms. Williams is willing to seek professional help. Billy, in spite of all the trauma and change, is doing well—he's not severely depressed, destructive, or oppositional. He can make friends, does well in the school structure, and must be fairly bright.

- *Therapeutic options*. Family therapy with Grandmother, Grandfather, Billy, and John to improve communication, define clear rules and roles, reduce stress, strengthen the hierarchy, explore loss, and develop support and nurturance for each of them. What about including Billy's mother and father in the family therapy to focus on loss, roles, support, coparenting? Or seeing Ms. Williams individually or together with her husband to order to work on parenting skills and help them manage Billy?

Perhaps supportive individual therapy with Ms. Williams would help her to reduce her stress and be better able to act more consistently with Billy. Psychological testing for Billy could be considered; it may serve as a quick way of assessing his personality and coping skills and isolating underlying emotional conflicts. Individual play therapy with Billy could help him work through his past trauma and grief, provide ongoing support, help him learn better ways of coping with his emotions, provide him with a positive male role model to offset the negative ones he has seen. Maybe some combination of all of the preceding.

- *Therapeutic don'ts*. Need to be sensitive to issues of abuse or abandonment. Don't want to overwhelm Grandmother.

- *Therapeutic dangers/countertransference issues*. Feeling angry or frustrated with Billy or his grandmother. Feeling overwhelmed or wanting to quit case. Feeling overresponsible for the family.

These last two points need some explanation. As mentioned earlier, the presenting problems and symptoms become broad working metaphors that can tell us what to avoid and where to be careful in our approach in order to prevent ourselves from becoming emotionally snarled within the system. Given Billy's history, we clearly know that he is sensitive to anger and aggression, from his experience with the boyfriend, and abandonment, from the loss of his parents, issues we need to keep in mind as we interact with him and plan his treatment. Similarly, because the grandmother is already feeling overwhelmed, we want to be careful that we don't do anything to make these feelings worse, nor replicate her own behavior and be inconsistent or unstructured in our approach; this will only further confuse her and leave her more inconsistent than she already is.

But this is only half the equation. Recognizing the subtlety and power of the dynamics means acknowledging that we too may be capable of feeling like the parents, or that we may get demanding, invasive, or insensitive to endings or breaks in contact. We may find reasons to send him off for individual therapy, or decide that the case and family are simply unworkable. Similarly, there is the danger that we may end up feeling like the grandmother—overwhelmed and willing to give in, feeling that we have to do it all on our own, overresponsible and exhausted.

By acknowledging the therapeutic dangers inherent in a particular case we are acknowledging the family and individual dynamics that can pull us like an undertow toward the replication of the family's problems, behavior, and emotions. Only by looking out for them, only by looking in and sensing when we emotionally are becoming ensnared, can we step back and regroup.

Again, at this point, we don't know how much of this will come to pass, and we need to assess Billy and his grandmother further. But through our brainstorming we have defined both our therapeutic possibilities and our limits. We have a clearer view of the therapeutic space we can work within.

OPENING MOVES

Some clinicians feel awkward about including children in family therapy. Two cultures, two different worlds, those of the children and those of adults, both need to be explored, understood, yet it's difficult. Parents feel they have to careful what they say around the children; children, especially if they are young, often feel intimidated by the office, by the questions, by the seriousness of all the talk that they don't understand. Like Billy, many children sense that they are in an adult place and grow quiet unless welcomed in some way. How you bring together these different worlds once again depends upon your theory and style. There is more than one path from which to choose.

Some clinicians prefer to see the parents alone first. This gives them a chance to gather background information about the problem, the child, and the marriage without the child distracting them or the parents feeling inhibited. They can vent and give details of their concerns without worrying about the child feeling the brunt of their criticisms. This adults-only meeting also binds the clinician to the parents more firmly, suggesting from the start a partnership among the adults. At the end of this session the clinician can then decide whether to see the identified child or the rest of the family, or perhaps even continue working with the parents themselves.

This parent-focused approach is particularly useful when the problem seems to be due to a simple lack of parenting skills or the parents' struggle and inability to form a united front. It's also useful when the parents expect that they only need to turn the child over to you to be fixed, when there is an adamant refusal of a teen to come to treatment, or when the overwhelming logistics make bringing in the entire family almost impossible. In all of these situations the clinician essentially sees how far he or she can get by empowering the parents and coaching them to be change agents in the home. Many times this is enough.

There are, however, two potential disadvantages to this format. The larger one is only seeing the problems through the parents' eyes; they may not be good reporters of the interactional patterns, or their concerns about "looking good" to you may severely slant their point of view. The other minor disadvantage is the awkwardness of bringing in the children later.

Generally it's best to start your relationship with young children by seeing them together with their parents. Have the parents describe why they came, clarify your role with the child (young children are often afraid that you are going to give them a shot like their pediatrician does), and get enough background to know what you want to explore with the child individually. As you talk together with the parents and child, the child will come to feel more comfortable with you, can get used to the sound of your voice, and can learn from watching the parents' reactions that you are a safe person. Then when you ask the parent to leave, the child will be less anxious and feel more comfortable staying with you. If the child balks at the idea of being alone with you, throwing him- or herself around a departing parent's ankle, don't force it; the goal of therapy is to reduce trauma, not create it. Let the parents stay for a while you when you begin to interact and play with the child.

For preteens or adolescents entering the second session, on the other hand, it's another story. They often feel mistrustful; they worry that unfair things have been said about them behind their back (and often they have), that the adults are plotting behind their backs and that you have taken their parents' point of view. While you can handle this straightforwardly and show your openness and sensitivity by simply asking them how they feel about missing the first appointment, or by spending enough individual time with them that they feel you understand their point of view and are unlike their parents in your reactions, you may have to work a little harder to gain their trust.

1st. session together

The classic family therapy approach, of course, is to see everybody in the family together the first session. The obvious advantage is your ability to see all the interactional patterns and roles at one time. You are able to shift the focus away from the I.P., and reinforce the notion that it is a family problem, a product of interaction, rather than the fault of the I.P. Pragmatically, total family sessions can make coming to the appointment easier; there's no need to worry about the expense and logistics of child care.

While total family sessions can be powerful, they can also feel overwhelming for you and the family: for you because of the number of people in the room, for them because they often have not sat together as a family in a long time and they are worried about your judgment or the exposure of secrets. It's helpful to keep in mind that you don't have to talk to the entire group all the time, nor do you need to do all the work. Talk to one person at a time, asking questions to gather the information that you need; allow everyone to have a chance to describe his or her view of the problem and feelings about being there. The goal is to help everyone feel safe through your leadership, your desire to understand their world, and your reassurance that they will not need to reveal anything until they are ready.

Direct them to talk with each other: "Mary, try telling your sister what hurt your feelings, rather than calling her names"; "Dad, tell Susan how you feel right now"; "Tommy, tell your mother why you think her rule is unfair." Block interruptions and make sure everyone gets a chance to speak. While the impulse to argue with each other can be strong, family members will quickly learn that the session doesn't have to degenerate into the big scene that it has so many times before. By discussing problems and emotions with each other right there in the session, they'll be doing more of the work, and you'll feel less stagefright and pressure to fix everything.

For families that are less reactive, more cautious, you goal is less maintaining control and more creating openness. Doing enactments with these families can warm them up to you and the therapy process, as well as give you more information about the process to which you can respond.

Your first couple of whole family sessions will seem the most difficult, so remember once again to be easy on yourself. With continued practice you'll get your sea legs, and it really will seem easier. If you feel stuck, remember to stay open and honest and go back to your basics.

Seeing Billy together with his grandmother (the grandfather was out of town) for the first session represented a middle ground between adults-only sessions and whole family sessions. While seeing the I.P., as I did, with one or both parents prevents you from seeing all the interactional patterns, you are able to nail down those surrounding the parent–child interaction. Working with this cluster can provide a starting point for your assessment and feel less overwhelming. Once you have a better lay of the land, you can then sort out who else to bring in or split up.

Whatever format you choose, even individual work with one parent, you are, of course, still doing family therapy if you're thinking systematically, that is, in terms of the family's interactional patterns. Calling yourself a family therapist isn't restricted only to those who pile 15 people in a room at one time.

While any of these formats can help you place the child and presenting concerns in the context of the family, the challenge usually remains, especially with young children, of how to more fully assess the child, how to enter his or her world when he or she may be overshadowed in the presence of parents or doesn't fully understand all the verbiage that's being tossed around. Some individual assessment is usually in order.

WORKING WITH PLAY

If fitting children into the family therapy process seems hard for some clinicians, the notion of play can seem even harder. Some clinicians simply don't feel comfortable with play as a therapeutic medium; they prefer words to crayons or blocks, the direct language of problem solving rather than the symbolic language of fantastical worlds within sand trays or playhouses. Others just don't feel comfortable around children—they don't have little ones of their own, or have had limited personal experiences in childhood, perhaps—and will choose either not to treat them at all, or to work through the parents. Still for others, the problem is largely one of their limited skill and experience; they simply haven't been trained in play therapy, are uncertain about the effectiveness, and struggle figuring out how to go about doing it.

Just as it's important to be aware of your own theory and values regarding your approach to families, it's important to be clear about your own approach to children. How do you feel about play therapy? Do you see it as a tool for assessment, treatment, or both? Do you view play as a potentially healing process in itself, or more an effective backdrop for talk therapy? When is it better to do individual play therapy than work with the parents, or with the child together with the parents? When is play therapy contraindicated? What about play therapy do you personally like or dislike?

Play, of course, is for children what words are for adults, namely, a medium of expression. Because they lack the vocabulary of an adult and a brain capable of creating the concepts and analogies that the adult mind can, children's words are often only flimsily attached to their thoughts and emotions. Rather than using language to express fantasies (looking forward to the big date on Saturday night), wishes (I wish my roommate was less critical), images (I could see myself exploding and quitting right there on the spot), the child is able to do the same through play. The family living in the playhouse always fight, and here comes the police officer to tell them to stop; the lion puppet tries to eat the mouse puppet and mouse runs and gets help from the zebra; the clay turns into a snake that slithers along around the outside of the bedroom and scares the little girl; the picture of the family leaves out the little brother, and the little boy is a tiny speck squashed between the two angry parents.

When five-year-old Jamie, sounding just like her mother, yells at the doll for not going to bed, she is expressing her needs and conflicts just as clearly, though more symbolically, as the adult who complains about the way her boss dumped on her once again. Your asking Jamie why she is so mad is no different than asking the adult why she feels like her boss is being so tough on her—all that is different are the media in which each relates.

What do you need to do play therapy? Not much. Crayons, paints, drawing paper, clay. Some blocks, a playhouse, people figures to live in the house, some cars, trucks, an ambulance perhaps. Puppets, animal figures, toy soldiers, some Legos. Board games—for younger children Uno, Candy-Land, Chutes and Ladders. For older ones checkers, Battleship, Risk, Sorry. Get a deck of cards, hook up a mini basketball net over your office door, use a Nerf ball for the basketball. Most of what you need to get started can be found in Wal-Mart, at garage sales, or from friends whose kids have outgrown their toys. Set them out in your office where the children can see them and choose them.

Apart from these larger issues of play therapy theory and techniques are the practical questions of using play therapy within the context of a particular family. Will this family, for example, support the play therapy process? Are they able to see it as a form of treatment rather than just play, or would focusing on their parental skills better meet their expectations and increase the chance for success? Are they, and you, willing to take the time needed to engage in what may be a slower process? Is there any danger of the child's I.P. status being reinforced through individual focus? Is the child a good candidate for play therapy?

If you identify yourself as a play therapist and view play therapy as a best practice model for treating children, this last question may seem foolish. While there are different theoretical approaches to play therapy, just as there are to adult therapy, there is no right way to play in play therapy, just as there is no right way to talk in adult therapy. You may be directive, for example, and offer specific games or toys to use, or suggest various scenes to play out. You then watch what enfolds, make reflective comments, label the child's emotions, perhaps encourage problem solving. If your style is nondirective, you may let the child choose whatever toys or games he or she wishes, observe the play, and occasionally say what you see the child doing and expressing.[1] Whatever the child does is information and grist for the mill. If the child refuses to play or plays in a seemingly closed and unproductive way (e.g., plays checkers for the whole session for 20 weeks), you still have clues as to how the child relates to adults or follows rules, approaches emotions or new situations, or competes against others or is able to be assertive, just as adults who seem sensitive to your comments, try and fill the space with small talk, or only occasionally grunt provide information about their interactional style.

While all this may be true, there remains the question of whether

[1]For additional information on play therapy theory and techniques, consult Eliana Gil, *Play in Family Therapy*, Guilford Press, 1994; Kevin O'Connor, *The Play Therapy Primer*, Wiley, 2000; Charles Schaefer, *Play Therapy Techniques*, Jason Aronson, 1994.

play therapy is a good match for a particular child and family. Just as some adults use one form of therapy more effectively than another, so too do children. Most children, for example, starting at age 10 or 11 on up, see any forms of imaginative play (the playhouse variety) as babyish. They would much prefer to talk, or use some structured play (e.g., board games, cards, basketball) as a background activity, a way of containing their anxiety while they answer questions or initiate conversation. Others do not want to play so much as hear their parents talk and have their questions answered, or, with your support, get things off their chests and solve problems at home or school. Still others are so reluctant or anxious about seeing you that the most effective and efficient course may be to work with the parents and effect changes at home through them.

What you actually wind up doing with children, then, is, as with adults, somewhere between the ideal and pragmatic, a blend of your comfortable media, needs, and style with theirs. For some children you may decide to use play therapy only as an assessment tool, a way of gathering information about the child that can then be passed on to the parents to help them view their child in a different light, or to help you develop behavioral strategies that the parents can implement at home. If, for example, you learn through his play that Bobby is worried about his parents divorcing, feels that he has to take care of his depressed father, or feels guilty about his younger sister's cerebral palsy, this information can help the parents be more supportive of Bobby or motivate them to talk to him about what has happened.

In another case it may be clear to you that play therapy may be the best not only for assessment but treatment as well. Only through the play process, for example, may the child be able to express many of the emotions that cannot be talked about directly. For example, Todd expresses his anger at his father by drawing a picture of him and then scribbling over and over it with a black crayon—anger that he is not able to express at home. For another child, what you do together doesn't really matter—playing the card game rummy this week, drawing pictures next week—but by playing together with you the therapeutic relationship becomes the support that allows the child to talk about his or her fears and worries. Just as you encourage adults to move against their grain and take risks, you do the same with the child in play. As the child becomes less anxious, more open, more confident, you may decide to intersperse total family sessions, involve other siblings in the play process, or work concurrently with the parents.

It's important to remember that the therapeutic contract is not only between you and the child, it's also between you and the parents. While some parents are too content to have you take over their child and treat him or her, often dangerously replicating their already ingrained hands-off stance, other parents can seem anxious or annoyed by what seems like a dark hole of individual play therapy. How you ultimately choose to work must reflect the parent's concerns and priorities as well. If, for example, they are particularly disturbed by the behavior of one of the children, spending a few sessions in the beginning in individual play therapy with that child, rather than pushing for family therapy, not only builds your own rapport with the child, but addresses the parents' immediate concerns. It gives you a stronger basis for recommending family therapy when you do—after all, you have "evaluated" the child, and have your own sense of what the child needs most. If, on the other hand, the family is in crisis, it may be better to begin with total family sessions, calming the emotional fires at home so they are less of a distraction before you shift to individual work with the child.

The bottom line here is that play therapy with children is another approach, another modality, another clinical choice. You can flexibly integrate it into your family therapy models and adapt to your own style and strengths, as well as the needs of particular child and family.

THE MORE THE MERRIER?: THE QUESTION OF MULTIPLE THERAPISTS

In sorting through treatment options, there is one final one to consider, namely, whether it's useful to divide a case and family among more than one therapist. The traditional child-study model favors this approach: A child specialist works with the child individually while another clinician works with the family. The classic family therapy approach is just to go ahead and see everyone.

Probably the worst basis for deciding this approach is convenience and logistics—you don't have time to see both the child and the family in the same week so you roped in a colleague to help out. This dismisses the clinical needs of the family. Some clinicians bring in another therapist as a way of offsetting their limited skills—rather than fumbling through play therapy, farm that individual work out to a specialist and turn your attention toward your strengths in family therapy—but this approach has to be weighed against the impact of multiple therapists on the family. Often it's better to do it all and increase the supervisory support and coaching. In other cases rapport or the lack of it is a deciding factor—the adolescent female, for example, could significantly benefit by some individual therapy to supplement the family therapy, but she has a strong negative transference to a male therapist. In that case, bringing in the female therapist to see her, and having both of you work together with the family may be the most prudent option.

Those clinicians who are uncomfortable with family work and think psychodynamically rather than systemically seem often to fall into a one problem–one therapist approach, with Mom, Dad, and the I.P. seeing separate individual therapists, then all coming together with a separate family therapist. I personally don't like this approach. Coordination among the therapists, which is essential, becomes difficult. There's the danger not only of confusion for the family members over how to integrate their different therapies or how to set priorities regarding goals, but also of clients splitting therapists—disclosing some information with one, some with another, deciding one is nurturing, the other cold and mean. In the worst-case scenario, all the therapists wind up replicating the family dynamics with confusion over who's in charge, fragmented focus, and squabbles over the treatment plan itself.

I prefer to do as much of the work myself as possible—not for control, but for consistency and coordination of the elements of the treatment plan. The family and I can cobble out one vision together that incorporates the overall needs of the family, rather than juggling several. There are a few exceptions. Sometimes I will farm out psychological testing to a psychologist for further assessment, but the boundaries are clear and his or her role stops at the assessment. If I believe a child may benefit from a medication evaluation, I will refer the family to a physician or psychiatrist, and coordinate so he or she is aware of my therapy goals and progress, and I can remain up-to-date about the medication. If I am struggling to build rapport with one of the key family members, I may consider bringing in a cotherapist to help out, for example, have a female therapist come in to support a mom who is the sole female in a family of males.

The only time I find myself clinically advocating for a separate therapist for one of the family members is when I think it is important to reinforce boundaries and underscore more clearly who is responsible for what problem. For example, if the father in a family tends to be abusive, I may suggest that he see someone separately to focus on his anger. Rather than seeing his anger as only a response to the rest of the family, this reinforces the notion of self-responsibility and self-regulation, and gives him the space to learn these skills, which can then be folded into the family work. Once again, the bottom-line criteria become moving toward what is missing and being careful not to replicate dysfunctional patterns. As with all the other clinical options, consider your own style and strengths and make your decision clinically based and intentional.

BREAKING GROUND: FIRST SESSIONS WITH THE CHILD

When a child remains quiet in the first session or two with parents, it's important to make the extra effort to connect with him or her. Because Billy was like this when I saw him together with his grandmother, I decided to meet with him for a few sessions alone to build rapport, find out better what he is like, and discover how he would use play therapy. Surprisingly, Billy was eager to be seen alone.

After glancing around the room, Billy makes a beeline for the Legos. He matter-of-factly tells me that he wants to build one of the models pictured in the instructions. It is clear that he can read well for his age, and has good spatial perception and coordination; he is much better figuring out how to do it than I am. He quickly begins to gather the pieces he needs and enlists my help in finding some of them, all with an air of seriousness and intensity. When I try to ask him about his coming to the agency, about living with his grandmother, about his father, his mother, he ignores the question, says he doesn't want to talk about it or says he doesn't know. He keeps all of his focus on the Legos and all of his communication limited to directing my help. At the end of the session, Billy hasn't finished his model, and he asks me to save it for next time. He wants to know when he is coming back.

The next several individual sessions aren't much different. Billy still talks little, though when asked he mentions without much enthusiasm that he saw his father over one weekend, and describes in a few sentences his school and teacher. When asked to draw his family he says that he doesn't draw people well, and when asked to draw anything else says he doesn't like to draw much. He does play Candy Land and tries to cheat when it appears he is going to lose. When I say that he isn't following the rules, he seems upset and reluctantly gives in. In the second game Billy makes up new rules as he goes along so that it always works to his advantage. Again his mood is fairly solemn, but he mentions several times that he likes to come and wants to know when he is coming back.

Impressions? What seems most striking is Billy's need for control of the session—directing me, controlling the conversation, controlling the outcome of games. What don't we see? What's missing? Obviously no strong emotions, like anger; no discussion about his past or the trauma; no aspect of his inner world, his fantasies; none of his misbehavior that his grandmother is reporting in the home. Billy isn't replicating his problems in the office. Why?

His behavior isn't surprising. Many children who have been traumatized have learned to cope by controlling themselves and others. They're both protecting themselves from other inner and outer dangerous emotions, and, on some level, replicating the control they experienced from powerful adults. Billy has learned that it's more important (and safer) to be in control than to be who he is. The only place he shows his emotions is at home with his grandmother. He probably trusts her enough to let down his guard, but he also may replicate with her the emotionality that he saw between his mother and father.

Is Billy a good candidate for play therapy? The answer lies in your orientation. As mentioned earlier, from a psychodynamic, more nondirective perspective it's a ridiculous question. If clients show up they're working in therapy, even if the working is both you slogging through all the defenses and layers of resistance. Billy is clearly showing up; in fact, he enjoys coming and likes me. At a minimum the relationship has the potential to give him an opportunity to be with a man who isn't abusing or rejecting, offsetting the male images he has within him.

The better question that a more directive therapist may ask is whether Billy is using the play therapy process effectively. The answer would probably be no. Compared to other children who start re-creating their inner and outer worlds from the start, Billy is not using the play as a medium for portraying his emotions and conflicts. Instead he's only showing his defenses, either because he's terribly closed to his inner life, still frightened of me, or both. What he's not doing is being resistant to the therapy process itself. Some children clearly don't want to be in the room, not because they are anxious about the process, but more because they are angry with their parents who made them come. They refuse to play or do so passive-aggressively. Billy is not like this; he is playing out his life. It's just going to take a while to reach the deeper layers of it.

What would you do? A fork on the path. Would you see him in play therapy, maybe have someone else see him individually, stick to family or parenting work? It might be good to see his grandmother before making any decision.

THE REST OF THE STORY: ASSESSING THE GRANDMOTHER

Ms. Williams comes in alone. Despite my efforts to reach to her husband, Ray, he is driving all over the state delivering supplies for a hardware store and is unavailable. Although it's just 11 in the morning, she already has that dog-tired look. After she got Billy off to school, she needed to stop by her parents' house to take them to the grocery store for a few things. After lunch she's going back to help her mother clean the house.

Ms. Williams talks easily. Billy seems to have settled down some in the past couple of weeks, but he still gives her a fit at times, especially in the past few days that Ray has been away. Although John, her son, is usually home in the late afternoon, he does little with Billy and does even less when she's having a hard time with him. She's not sure how much longer John will be staying with them; he keeps talking about moving out. She knows she ought to be more consistent with Billy, but his tantrums wear her out, and she starts feeling sorry for him. She finds herself making bargains with him all the time—bribing him with TV, treats from the store, desserts—if he'll clean up his room, finish his homework, not pester her in the grocery store. Sometimes it works, sometimes it doesn't.

Ms. Williams can easily talk about Billy's mother, about how she didn't like her from the start, how the mother dumped Ms. Williams's son Ed, Billy's father, for that lowlife who killed his own child. But she sounds more sad than angry. She also has mixed feelings about Ed: Maybe he's just having a hard time right now, she muses, maybe he will eventually take custody of Billy; two minutes later she says that she also knows that he really doesn't show any interest in the boy, that she ought just to realize that Billy will stay with her.

The overwhelming feeling in the room, however, is that she's overwhelmed. She is the caretaker of her immediate family and her family of origin. There's a history of depression in the family, and even though she shows no vegetative signs, it's easy to believe that she may get pretty depressed at times. She clearly seems committed to Billy and overall is doing fairly well, especially considering the fact that she is doing it all alone.

When asked what she wants, Ms. Williams says she needs help learning to be more consistent. She feels that it's good for Billy to see someone himself; she is still very worried about the effects of his brother's murder on him. She doubts that her husband will ever be able to come in and questions whether it would make any difference, since he is away from home so much.

Once again, impressions? An overworked grandmother with a good heart. A soft touch who has a hard time setting limits for both Billy and herself. She's motivated to work on her parenting, and that's certainly needed. She supports individual therapy for Billy, and it already seems to have a somewhat positive effect. What to do about Ray? Try harder to bring him in? Is it realistic if he really is away so much? What about her son John? If he is really going to move out, would it be better to help Ms. Williams be able to handle Billy on her own? What about Ed—is it possible to get him involved? Could Ms. Williams manage better if she were able to set limits in other areas of her life, such as with her parents, and reduce her stress?

We are at the first fork on the path. What to do? In situations like this it's helpful to look first at what the family is willing to do and weigh that against the possible results of pushing them to do something different. This family's motivation is for play therapy and individual help with parenting. In spite of Billy's control in the sessions, they seem, from his grandmother's report, to have a positive effect on his behavior at home. This may have to do with the process and therapeutic relationship, or with Ms. Williams's own decrease in anxiety now that someone is there to help her or help Billy deal with his past, or both. In the long run, of course, the play therapy ideally could become a flexible medium for unlocking Billy's emotions, and the consistency of a positive relationship may counter the negativity and loss of the past men in his life.

Only doing play therapy, however, would not be a good idea, I feel. Rather than bringing in the grandmother and other parental figures in Billy's life and helping them learn to relate better to him, there's the danger that I, as the individual play therapist, will, in effect, displace them, making what's already occurring worse. Even beginning play therapy, I realize that I need to be clear and certain about my commitment, especially if the process and progress will be slow. If I become too impatient I'll wind up replicating the problem and become another abandoning man in Billy's life.

Working with Ms. Williams alone, as she suggests, may help her set the structure Billy needs, reduce her anxiety, and increase her self-confidence. But like the play therapy, there are questions. Is it practical or foolhardy to believe that she can continue to carry the load of the families alone? Would individual work with her on parenting only maintain a potentially dysfunctional system? We may have to try and see. Sessions with Billy and his grandmother together at this early stage wouldn't seem promising—I could imagine it turning into complaints of the week, a lot of questions, silence from Billy, and to him only a milder form of verbal abuse. As he feels more secure and settled and begins to open up more, this format may become a positive option.

Your own theories may no doubt suggest other options: exploring with Ms. Williams her own depression, past losses, or the dynamics underlying her sense of overresponsibility; a parents' support group for Ms. Williams or a psychiatric evaluation for her depression; the use of a play therapy group or a battery of psychological testing for Billy. How about moving the therapy out to the home? A home-based therapist could see Billy and his grandmother there where the problems were occurring, give Ms. Williams hands-on demonstrations of parenting skills, have her observe and participate in the play therapy, and perhaps have greater success in pulling in Billy's uncle or grandfather. All of these are possibilities.

What was finally decided was the combination of individual play therapy with Billy and parenting education and support for Ms. Williams, a decision reflecting my own skills, interest, and orientations, the availability of services (home-based services, for example, had a huge waiting list), and the family's motivation and immediate needs. This plan was presented to both, Ms. Williams and Billy, and they seemed satisfied.

PUTTING THE PLAN INTO OPERATION

Over the next few months I saw Billy individually each week in play therapy, and saw his grandmother, either in individual sessions or for a few minutes at the start of Billy's session about every other week, to discuss parenting problems. Billy continued to need to control the session and resisted suggestions to engage in drawing, paints, storytelling, sand tray, clay, talking games, and other more expressive media.

The offering of play suggestions was, I felt, an important part of the process. Just as it's valuable to give adults a clear sense of the range of topics and forms that therapy may take, so is it important when working with children to help them see the range of what play therapy offers, and to find the medium that best suits the individual child. Some children, for example, love drawing or painting, but hate playhouses or board games. Others don't seem to care what the activity is. Many active children like to play outside, others seem attracted to the containment or regularity that the office session provides. It's up to you to introduce the choices and help the child discover the forms that allow him or her to express best his or her inner self.

Billy rejected all these less-structured forms because they created too much anxiety. He was able, however, gradually to express violent themes through playing with cars and trucks (creating gigantic crashes), toy soldiers where battles always ended with his army defeating mine, and—surprisingly—with wrestling.

Billy was a big fan of professional wrestling, and knew a lot about the different characters, their strengths and weaknesses, and, most importantly, whether they were good or bad guys. In a typical session he would move the furniture in the room to the corners, we would block the sharper corners of the furniture with cushions for safety, and Billy would assign me to be a particular "bad" wrestler—The Black Knight, Sergeant Destruction, Lowthar the Crusher—while he would always be the week's current world champion. We negotiated rules (e.g., where the ropes were, whether it was a tag team, how you were pinned, how long the match was) and they were restated and clarified at each session. Although Billy only weighed about 60 pounds, it was here that he became most animated and most aggressive, and where he always had to win. And he did; I made sure of it.

What's going on here, is this therapeutic? Doesn't this rough play only replicate the physical aggression he had already seen? Certainly—and that was the therapeutic rationale for doing it. Through the wrestling matches Billy was able to play out the anger that was being bottled up or dumped on his grandmother. He also was fighting with a big strong adult man, on some level not much different from the one who terrorized him. But now he had the opportunity to win. In his imagination he became powerful and able to overcome his enemies, rather than a helpless victim.

But he also had to learn to express aggression with constraint; the rules of the play included clear restrictions on aggression (you can't punch) and having to stop and let the other one up if either one of us felt hurt, tired, or uncomfortable. These rules taught Billy the beginnings of self-expression and self-control. Finally, this play provided Billy with a way of making physical contact with a man who, in reality, was not aggressive, but more nurturing. While he was pretending to pin me to the mat, he was, in actuality, getting hugged back.

All this raises the larger question of touch in therapy. As therapists we all have greater awareness of clients' possible past physical and sexual abuse than we may have had in the past; we know and are sensitive to the potential ethical dangers that physical contact can pose. Some therapists have moved toward feeling that any physical contact with clients is out of bounds. I tend to not be so austere. While we are thankfully way beyond the touchy-feely times of 30 years ago when everyone got a big hug or we justified clients sitting on our laps as part of a reparenting process, there are times when a pat on the back as a client walks out the door after a difficult session can physically give to a client what he or she can't yet psychologically give to him- or herself, when a gentle tap on the knee can be an effective nonverbal signal to a family member that he or she is once again getting hooked into a dysfunctional pattern and needs to resist the temptation.

Our ethical codes define clear bottom lines regarding physical contact, and our sensitivity to the client's history, experience, and reactions in the moment should serve as guides as to what we can or should not do when it comes to issues of touch. We should be clear about our clinical rationale based upon the client's goals and needs, be wary of rationalization, and be open to supervisory input when in doubt. But we should not, I believe, automatically dismiss the use of touch as a potential adjunct to talk therapy.

If I had initiated wrestling with Billy because I thought it was a good idea, rather than following his lead, he most likely would have simply gone along. But emotionally this would have been potentially injurious to him because we would have succeeded in replicating his powerlessness, as well as potentially triggering old emotional and physical reactions. If I had failed to set rules and literal boundaries, or had not ensured that he was safe, or had ignored his own limits, I would have once again repeated in minor form the neglect that he had previously experienced. But I was following his lead, working within his metaphors, and the wrestling became an outlet for his emotions, an opportunity for self-mastery and self-regulation, a chance for him literally to rewire the meaning of touch.

MAKING PROGRESS?

Billy settled down more and more at home and, with support from me, Ms. Williams was able to set clearer limits. She used time-outs and taking away of privileges, along with verbal positive reinforcement to shape Billy's behavior at home. Within five months the presenting problem—Billy's testing of limits at home—had waned considerably.

But not all the time. Here and there were periods of a week or two where things would slip at home: The grandmother was less consistent with the rules, the structure began to collapse, Billy started pushing, and the grandmother gave in, setting off a self-feeding cycle. From the grandmother's point of view it was Billy who started the backsliding process—for some reason he had a hard day or week and would test her. From where I stood it was Ms. Williams who actually started the cycle. Some additional outside stress would stretch her psychological resources, and she was unable to maintain her consistent focus on Billy.

Within the five months several environmental disruptions and emotional crises had occurred—Ray was unemployed for several weeks before he found another job, John was having problems with his ex-wife and getting depressed, Ms. Williams was worried about her father, who was having pain in his hip and needed to go to the doctor. As the stress increased and Ms. Williams became more worried, upset, and depressed, she let things go, opening the door for Billy to return to his older behaviors, and further increasing her own stress. As the problems resolved—for example, when Ray found a job—the structure returned.

What sense do you make of this dynamic? Do the new parenting skills collapse in the face of stress because they are still fragile and not well integrated? Does Ms. Williams's chronic depression grind her to a halt when the stress is high enough? Does Billy become defiant as a way of getting his grandmother's attention when she seems preoccupied and he starts to feel abandoned, or is he perhaps trying to save his grandmother, attempting to pull her out of her depression by his negative behavior, and replicating what he did with his mother? Is he needed as a problem at these times because he also provides an outlet for his grandmother's or the family's frustration and anger? Has he learned to sacrifice himself as the scapegoat?

All of these are possible ways of looking at the pattern, and they're important only in the way they help you proceed. Once again consider the options and your own inclinations. Would you support Ms. Williams in staying on track with the parenting, perhaps interpret to her Billy's behavior and role in the family based upon his past experience? Would you advise her about how to solve the problems at home, realize the limits of her own responsibility, offer support or specific skills (e.g., teach relaxation exercises) to help relieve her anxiety, refer her for medication? Would you bring in Ray or John, or both, to get to the source of the stress, and use the crisis as an opportunity to get them involved in the family therapy process? Would you do something different with Billy perhaps, increasing the frequency of his sessions, or working to help him express his anxiety verbally rather than behaviorally?

All of these are workable. You could try one of these, several, something all together different, or decide that these changes are, for right now at least, merely a blip and do nothing different at all.

I decided to do something else. In situations like this it's often useful to go back and look at what's working and to find ways to support those processes. Overall, the current approach of doing play therapy with Billy and focusing on parent education and support with Ms. Williams was creating stability at home and improvement in Billy's behavior. It didn't work when the stress became too great for Billy's grandmother. If there was a way of reducing her overall level of stress, then crises, when they arose, would debilitate her less, and, I reasoned, she would be able to continue to maintain the structure that Billy needed. Pulling in Ray or John, or helping Ms. Williams find ways to reduce the responsibilities she had with her parents all theoretically have the same impact, but practically speaking, weren't, in her view or mine at the time, good options. Trying to make such changes would be enormously difficult (so who would help the parents?) and would undoubtedly create even more stress, only compounding the problem.

And so I supported her in maintaining the behavioral structure as much as possible (the redoing and reinforcing that is part of the middle stage), and emotionally by simply listening to her. I also arranged respite care for Billy a few days a week after school and on alternate weekends, an idea that both Billy and his grandmother thought was great. Here he would spend time with another family, one that was part of the community respite program. This program arose out of the community need to help overloaded parents of physically and mentally disadvantaged children, as well as families like Billy's, by giving them a break from a few hours to a couple of days at a time, on a regular basis.

As it turned out, the respite family that was assigned to Billy had two boys around Billy's age. The family did a lot of activities (soccer, camping) that Billy didn't get to do at home, and the parents in the family were both supportive and good at limit setting, exactly what Billy needed. Ms. Williams appreciated the break, and Billy not only enjoyed the time there, but found that he could separate from his grandmother and she and he would be all right.

It helped. As the crises came and went, both Billy and his grandmother were able to step outside them a bit better. More importantly, Ms. Williams was better able to see the connection between her stress and Billy's reaction, and could even anticipate the start of the negative cycle; his behavior was less and less seen as arbitrary or instigating. All the pieces seemed to be coming together.

Looking Within: Chapter 9 Exercises

1. In considering the initial assessment of Billy and his family, what most strikes you as important to focus upon? What therapeutic options would you choose based upon your style and theory?

2. What are your own feelings and thoughts about the use of touch in therapy?

3. All children engage in play as a means of understanding and coping with the stresses of their world. When you look back on your own childhood, what type of play was most prevalent? What themes continued to run through your play even as you grew older? What do you think they may say about your stresses and needs?

[10]

Billy

THE STORY CONTINUES

IN THE MIDDLE OF THE MIDDLE

As we discussed in Chapter 7, the middles of treatment are a time of developing skills and reinforcing changes (in infinite variations it seems) over and over again until they can be permanently integrated into the family's patterns. The middle stage can also be a time when the focus of treatment will shift; Once the child problem is settled, the marital issues come to the surface; now there is time and trust in the therapeutic relationship to explore a parent's individual concerns, such as his or her own past history of abuse, of depression, or of problems with sex or drugs. After a quick start, individual sessions with the child may seem to level off and show little movement, but crises may break out elsewhere in the family as the still-active dysfunctional patterns are pushed in new directions. A shift to parent sessions to firm up skills may be more productive, or, if the child has become stronger and articulate through individual work, it may be a good time to focus on family sessions.

Billy slowly progressed during this middle time. While he stayed relatively closed to his past, he did begin to let go of his need to be in charge. In sessions he no longer needed to direct me. My relationship with him, based on being absolutely predictable and reliable, increased his sense of trust. He was able to compromise; he was more sensitive to my feelings; his play themes became less violent. Wrestling, once so intense, became more of an occasional thing. At home Ms. Williams was by and large able to maintain the structure that Billy needed, and, with the help of regular respite, things generally went smoothly. But then everything became unsettled once again—the parents came back in the picture.

Although Billy's mother hadn't seen Billy for two years and had no contact beyond a couple of letters, she now started writing, telling him that she wanted to come visit. Ms. Williams would come into sessions waving letters, wondering what to do, how to respond, to Billy, to his mother. She had fantasies of his mother taking Billy away, of her filling his head with something (she didn't know what) about the past, and causing him to regress back to where he started. Why couldn't she, the grandmother wondered aloud, just leave him alone?

The grandmother's reaction wasn't unusual. Anytime an absent parent comes back into a child's life, for both the child and the caretaker it creates anxiety that can disrupt the system. For Ms. Williams the mother became a threat: Even though the grandmother had legal custody, the mother was his mother, and could, it seemed, take him back if she wanted to. Making it all the worse, of course, was Billy's reaction. He idealized his mother and was excited about the prospect of seeing her again.

Ms. Williams realized she couldn't stop the visits without court action, but she decided that there needed to be some supervision, and so she drafted some additional relatives to be around when the mother came. I asked about Billy's mother coming to a session—this would not only provide a safe forum for meeting and talking, but would give me an opportunity to see this other important person of Billy's life up close—but no, the grandmother replied, his mother was planning on coming on Sunday only for a few hours.

But the mother didn't come. No phone call. No letter, nothing. Fortunately, the grandmother and I had discussed this possibility. Ms. Williams was both relieved and angry. Billy said little. Ms. Williams was tempted to use this incident as an example to show Billy just what kind of person his mother was, but I tried to help her see that this was her agenda, her emotions, very separate from Billy's own. He needed the opportunity to deal with his grief himself and to come to terms with his mother and their relationship without the grandmother injecting her own feelings. I tried to talk to Billy about it, made interpretative comments about how he might feel—angry and sad, that she really didn't care, that there was something wrong with him—and offered to help him write a letter to his mom. In typical Billy style, he remained closed and quiet.

On the heels of this incident reentered Billy's father, Ed. A shadowy and sporadic presence, he too suddenly expressed an interest in seeing Billy more, even talked to Ms. Williams about taking custody. Why all the renewed interest wasn't clear; Ms. Williams suspected that it had something to do with his stable relationship with his girlfriend. Because it was her own son, she felt less threatened, but only slightly. She quickly made clear to Ed that Billy (and she) could not handle any whimsical or quick changes. If he was serious about custody, he could prove it by visiting regularly, and everyone would see how things went over the course of a year.

Billy was less excited about his dad's visits. The parents had divorced when Billy was two years old, so his memories of his father were nonexistent, and his experience with him since he had been with his grandmother had been disappointing. Again I invited the father into session, but he said he worked long hours and couldn't get the time off. The father began weekend visits, but after a month started to find reasons not to come. Within two months he had stopped seeing Billy altogether.

This kind of in-and-out involvement can be devastating for a child. The child has no stable relationship on which to lean; he literally becomes afraid to open his heart. The rejections are a narcissistic injury, proving that he is unlovable, which can cause depression and rage. It also can be infuriating for you as a therapist. It's difficult not to identify with the child, and, like the grandmother, be angry at the parent and project your reactions onto the child. But while your own countertransference can give you a clue to how the child may be feeling, your focus is on helping the child sort through his or her own grief reaction.

Billy remained stable for a few months in spite of these rejections, but then the stronger emotions began to surface. His mother wrote another letter, and Billy refused to look at it. When Ms. Williams pressed it on him, he tore it up. He started having tantrums again at home when he couldn't get his way with his grandmother, and often refused to go into time-out when he misbehaved. Finally, there was an incident at school where a child pushed him on the playground and he attacked the child with such ferocity that it took three teachers to pull him off. He kicked one of the teachers so hard that he cracked her leg bone.

But the deterioration didn't stop there. His classroom behavior became increasingly oppositional, culminating two weeks later in another outburst where he turned over all the desks in the room. Now not only was Ms. Williams in a panic, so was the school administration.

In individual sessions Billy said little, and behaved no differently, but in a joint session with Billy and his grandmother, she repeated what Billy had told her—that the boy on the playground reminded him of Tom, the mother's boyfriend. This is a classic posttraumatic stress trigger, and what eventually came out of the session, with questions and prodding by both the grandmother and me as Billy sat on the floor near my chair, were Billy's memories of his brother's death—his hearing the commotion in his brother's room, his own fear about what was happening, the screams of alarm by the mother, the police. Most of all he remembered Tom blaming him for his brother's death.

The memories and the emotions were finally breaking loose. It may have been triggered by the reappearance and subsequent reabandonment by the parents, the lowering of his own defenses through therapy, the increased sense of safety by the grandmother's consistent presence and structure, the passage of time, a combination of all of them, or none of the above—it's difficult to really know. But what was clear was that he was beginning to process his trauma, and the emotions surrounding it were coming to the surface. What he needed most was support to verbalize these feelings, adequate channels for expressing them, and help understanding what was true and what was not.

What was not true, of course, was that Billy was responsible for his brother's death. As happens for many abused children, words heard in the moment became indelibly linked to the traumatic experience itself.[1]

Tom's accusation had stayed with and had haunted Billy for all those years.

It's tempting as the clinician to jump in and simply say to Billy that Tom was wrong and that he wasn't to blame. While intuitively this seems to make sense and, in cognitive-behavioral terms, corrects the cognitive distortion, this kind of response can feel like a too-quick, flip dismissal that has little absolving effect. Unless Billy had the opportunity to say why *he felt* he was to blame, that feeling and the idea would continue to stay within him. By our questions and listening his grandmother and I needed to let him know that we understood how he felt.

---

[1]For further information on treating children with trauma and attachment disorders, see Eliana Gil, *The Healing Power of Play*, Guilford Press, 1991; Nancy Boyd Webb, *Play Therapy with Children in Crisis*, Guilford Press, 1999; Richard Kagan, *Rebuilding Attachments with Traumatized Children*, Haworth Press, 2004; Terry Levy, *Attachment, Trauma, and Healing*, CWLA Press, 1998; Nancy Thomas, *When Love Is Not Enough: Families by Design*, 1997.

I asked if he sometimes felt that Tom was right, that it was his fault. He nodded. Did he think he should have done something different? Slowly, in half sentences and mumbles, he said that he felt that he should have somehow stopped Tom. How? I asked. He shouldn't have listened to his mother—he should have left his room, hit Tom maybe, tried to pick up his brother and run away into the back woods. Something. He teared up. He said he felt mad at himself for not doing anything.

As he spoke we both listened and restated and sympathized with his feelings. His grandmother held him. We then both reassured him as other adults who knew him and cared about him (in contrast to Tom who didn't) that it truly wasn't his fault. This seemed to calm Billy. As we were walking back down the hall after the session the grandmother said that now that lid seemed to be off the box, so to speak, she worried that Billy would continue talking about this at home and that she wouldn't know the right thing to say. I told her that she just needed to let him know that it was all right to talk about all this as he needed and wanted to and that she only had to listen.

But Billy didn't talk any more about this at home, and it seemed as though a breakthrough had been made. Later that week, however, he had another, seemingly unprovoked, outburst at school. The school principal arranged a meeting of all the people working with Billy.

COORDINATION WITH SCHOOLS

School behavior and performance are an important part of your assessment of a child or adolescent. The perspective of teachers, guidance counselors, and the principal can help you gauge how widespread particular problem behaviors may be, how the child responds in a setting different from home. Billy, for example, traditionally did well at school, as well as at camp and the respite home, environments where the structure remained consistent. School, in fact, for Billy and many other children, often becomes a place of important regularity and emotional security.

But it also possible for home and school to become emotional dumping grounds for each other. Some children are quiet and well-mannered at school, but belligerent at home. The home may be a safer, more secure place for the child to be him- or herself, or a place where trials and traumas of school life (being teased or picked on by other children, feeling criticized or castigated by a teacher, feeling embarrassed or shy) get acted out. Other children expend a lot of energy "holding it together" at school and emotionally collapse once they hit the door.

For some the pattern is reversed. The child that is perfect at home may be a holy terror in the classroom. Sometimes this reflects the home's low expectations of behavior—the child can essentially do whatever he or she wants, and rebels under the rules and regulations of the classroom—but more often it's the case that the home is not a safe place to show anger. The child copes at home by stifling strong emotions and uses school as an arena for releasing them. A positive change at one site may or may not create positive changes at the other. It's good to check and see whether a child is truly integrating changes and improving across settings.

It also important to see if the home and school are working together. Oftentimes they are not. While the school personnel are ideally concerned about the welfare of the whole child, in more pragmatic terms they're most concerned about the child as a learner. If the child is a good student, completes the work, and keeps his or her hands to him- or herself, underlying emotional issues can be easily ignored. When the child refuses or stops learning, bothers other children, or becomes a distraction in the class, as Billy did, the school sees a major problem, and at this point may refer the child for counseling. The school is essentially having a problem which the parents or child may or may not see.

This was the case now with Billy. The school teacher and administration were frightened by this 60-pound boy, by his rage, by his unpredictability. Unlike some other schools, they had no protocols for handling children like this, no organized response, such as time-out or restraints, to such behavioral or emotional outbursts. Instead, they reacted differently each time, and often, in their seeming panic, overreacted. One time as Billy flung desks around the room the teacher cleared all the other children out and watched through the window in the door until uniformed police finally arrived; their response unknowingly re-created Billy's past.

In large multidisciplinary meetings with school personnel the therapist has several tasks, depending upon the particular child and circumstances. Sometimes his or her job is simply to be present as an advocate or support to the parent who has clear ideas of what he or she wants for the child, but who feels intimidated by all the heavyweight professionals sitting around a table. Other times the school wants input from the therapist about the counseling, insights the therapist may offer in formulating a plan for the child at school; the therapist is often in a unique position to serve as a bridge between home, school, and office, providing a unified point of view for managing the child. What the school personnel generally don't want is the therapist criticizing their efforts, or telling them, unless they ask, what they should do. Their goals and needs for the child may be very different than those of the therapist, and like the therapist and the parent, they too feel they are doing the best they can.

So what could I say about Billy? At the start of therapy I had secured signed releases from the grandmother and Billy to talk with the staff at the school, and had already talked to Billy's teacher, guidance counselor, and principal several times in past months. At the meeting, with the grandmother present (Billy occupied himself in the nearby computer lab), I reviewed the history of my work with Billy: how he had responded to play therapy over the course of almost a year, about his need for control and the gradual easing up of these defenses, of the grandmother's work in providing a more structured environment at home, which Billy needed to feel safe. I also told them, with Ms. Williams adding details along the way, about Billy's recent experience with his parents, and the disclosure of his memories about both his brother and the abusing boyfriend. Finally, I said that I thought that Billy was actually getting better and beginning to heal. His recent behavior, though disruptive, was linked to the release of anger and grief that Billy had kept such a tight hold on for years.

While this last point was initially hard for some of the school staff to accept, when heard in the light of Billy's history and with my interpretations, they were able to agree. Framing these changes as positive gave the school personnel a new perspective, as well as helped them be more sympathetic to Billy's situation. Hearing this summary helped the grandmother realize just how far Billy had come.

But do you agree with my interpretation? If you were working with a child who presented with minor behavior problems, had been traumatized early in life but expressed little about his experience in therapy, and now began to have emotional outbursts and destructive behavior, would you think he was really making progress (things have to get worse before they get better approach) or would you think, based upon your theory and perspective, that he is really beginning to fall apart? What recommendation would you make to the school?

Regardless of the way Billy's new, aggressive behavior may be interpreted, it clearly could not be ignored. A different response and plan of action was required. We are at another fork on the path. Some questions and options to consider:

- Is it true that the school environment is no longer able to support him? Given the structure of the classroom and the demands on the teachers, would school become in reality only an arena for his negatively reinforced destructive behavior and deteriorating social relationships and self-esteem?
- What specific changes could and should the school make that might make a difference?
- Would he do better in a school setting that was more structured or geared for children with emotional problems, or would he, in fact, do worse, because of the stress of the change and the influence of potentially more negative role models?
- Would such a placement be premature? Would it represent a falling into the trap anticipated at the start, namely, a replication of the multiple abandonments he experienced with his parents?
- Should I, as the therapist, do more—increase sessions, take a more directive approach, secure some sort of evaluation or consultation? Should medication, in spite of his young age, be considered?

Difficult choices. Success, it seemed, depended upon what the school could tolerate and provide in the way of a positive response and services; upon Billy's ability to verbalize, rather than act out his anger and sadness; and the length of time it might take for him to work through his grief and anger and become less explosive.

What was finally decided at the meeting was that the school staff would try and put more emphasis on prevention. They were not comfortable using any form of restraint, but they would more closely monitor Billy's behavior over the course of the day and offer support—the teacher would check in with him and see how he was feeling, especially when he seemed irritable; she would take time to help him talk about and solve his problems with other children. Because he seemed to have the most difficulty in the afternoon, Billy would be given supervised individual computer time both as a way of reducing his afternoon stress and as a reward for good behavior. Finally, the school psychologist agreed to meet with Billy weekly for a half hour to further shore up problem solving and support within the school.

It seemed like a good plan and everyone around the table felt optimistic. It seemed to dovetail well with the home and therapy goals—developing consistent supportive but structured environments, helping Billy verbalize rather than act out his emotions—while I would continue to address the underlying grief and anger in play therapy. After the meeting, Billy's teacher, grandmother, and myself met with him to explain the school changes, and I followed up when I saw him at the next therapy session. Billy seemed fine with the plan.

But the changes didn't hold. After a honeymoon period of a few weeks, Billy exploded one morning when the teacher wouldn't let him get up to sharpen his pencil. The school administration once again panicked, and this time suspended him. They refused to allow him back into school until further evaluation could be done. I made arrangements for Billy to spend two weeks on the children's ward of the local private hospital.

NEW EYES, NEW IDEAS

While it's hard not to see a sudden hospitalization in the middle of therapy as cause for disappointment, I thought the school's idea to get a thorough evaluation done was a good one. The old dynamics were beginning to be played out—the emotional explosions on both sides, the cutoffs, the potential abandonment. Two weeks would give everyone a respite, a chance for regrouping and recharging. Through the workup some new information and recommendations might come out. Having someone with new eyes see a client, whether it be on an outpatient or inpatient basis, can be invaluable for overcoming the blind spots that can develop over time, for reaffirming what you know, or for providing a new perspective that can generate new ideas.

As could be predicted, Billy did well in the hospital. Once again the tight structure decreased his negative behavior, and group therapy with other children his age helped him to be more verbally open about his feelings overall. While he didn't talk much about his brother, father, or mother, he willingly participated in all the activities, kept a journal, and was able to make brief comments about his past to various staff. Both the grandmother and I made separate visits to see Billy at the hospital, in an effort not only to see how he was doing, but to maintain the reliability and predictability of his relationships, and reduce the sense of abandonment.

Some useful information and changes did come out of Billy's stay in the hospital. Thorough psychological testing confirmed a diagnosis of posttraumatic stress disorder and depression. The evaluators agreed that his recent explosive behavior was a result of a relaxation of his defenses through therapy and a relatively more stable home life; they suggested that the therapy continue as it was. Billy was placed on imipramine to relieve his depression and clonadine to reduce his aggression. But it was the formal reporting of the findings by the hospital psychologist and psychiatrist to the family—grandmother, grandfather, and John, Billy's at-home uncle—that had the most impact, especially upon both the men.

Consultations are often valuable not only for what they offer in terms of information, but also for who delivers it and how. In this case the clout of the psychologist and psychiatrist in their white coats in a wood-paneled office carried authority that I as the therapist could never match. The evaluation, the testing, the medication sent a clear message to these men that Billy truly had serious problems and needed their help. (Of course, in a different setting with a different family this could backfire—the medication becomes proof that the child is the only one with the problem, and reinforces his or her role of scapegoat.) With my prompting, the psychologist and psychiatrist strongly encouraged the men of the family to become more involved and back up Ms. Williams as much as possible.

The confrontation had an effect. When Billy went home a few days later there was renewed energy in the family. John, in particular, not only supported his mother when she set limits with Billy, he started taking a more active interest in him, playing catch in the evening, helping Billy with his homework, stepping into a paternal role. Although the school administration kept their fingers crossed, knowing Billy was now on medication, they took him back in. His teacher reported that he seemed calmer, steadier in his mood, and better able to do his work.

Often there's a honeymoon effect after a hospital stay. With the respite, new information, or change in treatment, the fact that the child is discharged (and therefore medically certified as better), it's easy for everyone to have renewed optimism. The problem is, of course, that all this optimism can wear off in a matter of days and, now that the "hospital solution" has become a solution, it's tempting for parents to bounce the child right back if things start to slide back downhill.

Such transition problems become even more difficult when a child has been in the hospital for several weeks or months. Like the family of the sailor or soldier who may be out of the home for months at a time, the family with the hospitalized child learns to reshape itself around the hole created by the child's absence. The parents have forgotten just how time consuming the child really is, or how quickly tension and triangles can build, or another child has been able to slip in to take up a lot of Dad's attention that used to go to the hospitalized child. Faced with the challenge of the returning child and the need for the family to create a new role for the child, it often unfortunately is easier for everyone to just let him or her fall back into the old one.

CALLING IN REINFORCEMENTS

Such falling back happened to Billy, but not for lack of trying. Crises once again began to brew—Ms. Williams's father fell down and hurt his leg, her husband was laid off again from his job at the hardware company, and John's five-year-old son came to stay for a few weeks while his mother was in the process of moving.

Everything fell apart. Now that John was spending free time with his son, Billy resented the cousin and all the attention he was receiving. Even though the grandfather was now around the house more, the noise and commotion created by the additional grandson, as well as his own depression around his job loss, made him irritable and withdrawn. And Ms. Williams, who had been doing much better with the support she was receiving, once again became overwhelmed, anxious, and depressed. Billy once again became more demanding, and grandmother once again caved in and gave in. The structure began to collapse.

The deterioration at home spilled over to school. Although there were no explosions, Billy began to act up. He talked back to his teacher, argued with other children, wasn't completing his work. The school went back to Plan A with the weekly meetings with the psychologist and afternoon computer time. This seemed to take the edge off, and gave the school some sense of control. In therapy Billy was able to talk about his jealousy and resentment of his cousin—a remarkable achievement for this silent child. I supported the grandmother and grandfather and worked with them to solve problems and stop the backslide, but neither one could really get mobilized. In order to avoid another hospitalization, I decided to call in reinforcements.

Home-based services were started to supplement the office-based therapy. Twice a week, for two hours at a time, a female therapist went out to the home to help the grandmother and grandfather (when he was around) manage Billy in specific situations. It was hands-on, primarily coaching the grandmother on the setting of limits and the implementing of time-outs. She also met with John and encouraged him to keep up his relationship with Billy, as well as back up his mother. Finally, the home-based worker served as a support for Ms. Williams, providing her with an opportunity to talk to about the stresses and strains she was experiencing. Although the family was cool at first about having this stranger in their home, they quickly warmed up to her. To provide even more support to Billy and the family, Billy's respite care with the other family was also increased.

But it wasn't enough. Even though Billy continued to use his individual sessions productively—both playing out and talking about his anger at the cousin, the abandonment by the uncle, his worries about his grandmother—and actually behaved well for a day or two after a session, he couldn't maintain it for more than that. Neither could the rest of the family. Within a few hours after the home-based therapist left, Ms. Williams or the grandfather would undo everything the clinician tried to reinforce. Even when John's son returned home to his mother and some of the stress was reduced, the structure in the home remained weak.

Billy had another explosion at school that came seemingly out of the blue. He punched a boy and bloodied his nose, slipped out of the teacher's grip when she tried to stop him, kicked her, and then ran out of the school and hid in some bushes off the school property. The police were called, and it was they who found him.

Billy was expelled. The school administration would provide home tutoring for the remaining three months of the school year. Now that he was home all the time, his grandmother was frantic. Both Ray and John were working temporarily on full-time jobs, and she was stuck home with Billy all day long. He pushed at her, and she invariably gave in just to get some peace.

Another crossroads. Once again several therapeutic options open up. Should individual therapy for Billy, for Ms. Williams, or home-based services be increased? Send him back to the hospital, have his medication reevaluated? Maybe just wait it out? Again it depends on how you see the problem. How much did the presence of the other grandson re-create and refuel Billy's own dormant feelings about his younger brother? (I tried to pursue this with him but got nowhere.) Is the chaos and abandonment, this time by the school, increasing Billy's anxiety and fears? How much of Billy's behavior is the product of the family dynamics, where Billy is so entrenched in his role, where the grandmother is so overwhelmed and her potential supports so unavailable?

All the professionals who were involved with Billy—me, the home-based therapist, school principal, special education coordinator, school psychologist, respite care coordinator—met with the grandparents to consider these questions and options. The consensus was that we had probably reached the limits of what outpatient services could do. We recommended placing Billy in a specialized residential treatment center for at least six months. Here he could attend school in a setting that could appropriately respond to his behavior (small classes, token economy, use of time-outs and restraints if needed). He would get individual and group counseling, and ideally have a chance to focus and work more intensively on his past trauma and loss, develop his social skills, and learn more effective ways of handling his emotions. The center we had in mind was close enough that the family could visit as his earned privileges would allow, and the overall plan was to gradually increase visitation stays as time of discharge became closer.

We also thought it would be best for the home-based therapist to continue to come once a week to do family therapy. Both she and I felt that the environmental and emotional problems within the family, if not alleviated, would undermine the structure Billy would need even after discharge. Ms. Williams's depression needed to be addressed, probably through medication, perhaps with individual therapy or marital therapy as well, and the men in the family needed to change their role and become consistently involved in parenting if Billy was going to be able to grow up in their home. Finally, as a way of maintaining our relationship, keeping a check on his progress, and offsetting his sense of abandonment, Billy would continue to see me two times a month. In order to facilitate coordination and treatment planning, everyone was to meet with the facility staff on a regular basis.

The family and I felt both failure and relief at this decision. On one hand the initial goal of not abandoning Billy seemed betrayed—the boy was to be sent away, replicating another loss, another desertion by the adults in his life. On the other hand, time was running out. The next year or two would, in my mind, be crucial in Billy's development. Unless he was able to grieve his losses, heal the trauma he experienced, and find healthier ways to express his emotions, his current behavioral patterns could solidify, increasing the risk that he could, like his mother's boyfriend, become dangerously violent. The grandparents, too, looked ahead with anxiety. Unless Billy could learn to manage his emotions and behavior or they could learn to better handle him, he would, as an adolescent, easily spin out of control.

Of course, Billy had his own mixed feelings. The grandparents and myself told him that the move wasn't because he was bad or being punished, but because we were having trouble giving him all the help that he needed. We wanted him to be able to go to school (something he wanted very much), rather than stay at home, and this seemed the best way to do it. We told him the plan for visits with the grandparents and me. He seemed excited about all the activities that the center provided, and knowing that he would be seeing and talking to everyone on a regular basis seemed to reduce much of his anxiety.

Although Billy had a difficult adjustment at first, he settled in within a couple of months and quickly moved up their level system. Although he did not talk much in individual therapy, he did open up in group—there were a couple of other children who had lost parents through death or divorce, and this helped him talk about his own feelings. When he came home on weekend visits, he seemed to the grandparents to be better behaved and more open. When he came to see me, we primarily spent the time catching up and playing games—more relationship maintenance than any therapeutic exploration.

The family procrastinated on seeing the home-based therapist, and this contributed to an extension of Billy's stay at the center by an additional five months. Part of this procrastination came from the family's need to have a break from focusing on problems. Part was probably due to their difficulty understanding how talking about parenting would be helpful if Billy wasn't there to create problems, and a good part was their own anxiety about stirring the family pot and talking about family problems that weren't specifically tied to Billy.

Like most families who have focused their attention on the problems of one child, Billy's absence made them more acutely aware of what else was wrong in the family. Without the ability to use Billy as a familiar distraction, they became more aware of the tensions, the problems, and their first reaction was to ignore the whole thing.

But the home-based therapist persisted. Just as the family members needed to learn how to interact with each other without Billy being in the center of them all, they need to learn how to interact and trust the home-based therapist without exclusively focusing on Billy and his problems. It took a lot of reassuring by the therapist, a lot of interpreting and normalizing of how they might be feeling, a lot of explaining over and over again the connection between Billy's long-term improvement (and coming home) and their ability to change the way the family operated.

It took Ms. Williams almost four months to go to the doctor and start on the Prozac that the doctor prescribed. It took more than five months before the couple consistently would meet for couple therapy. Family sessions with John were eventually included when the marital issues spilled over or when there was a need to talk about parenting issues.

Billy is back in public school and doing well. He continues to check in with me once a month or so, and because of the skills he learned at the center and the fact that he's getting older, we talk more now and play less. He still has no contact with his parents, but he is able more and more to look at those relationships as a reflection of them and not himself. Although he's put much of his past behind him, losses (the death of his dog, his uncle moving away for a few months) spark his defiance and irritability, test his grandparents' ability to maintain their limits, and stir memories of his brother's death.

While the present seems stable, the risks for the future are still there. His grandparents had trouble in adolescence with all their children, and while their awareness and parenting skills have increased, the danger of sliding back into those patterns remain. It's made all the worst by the simple fact that the grandparents are getting older. They may physically find it more and more difficult to keep up with a growing adolescent.

The normal ups and downs of adolescence are right around the corner for Billy. As is typical for teenagers who have been abandoned by their parents, Billy's feelings about his parents—anger at their neglect, curiosity about what they are like—will undoubtedly come to the surface. These feelings in turn will drag up the unresolved past all over again—his wondering what's wrong with him, his guilt over his brother's death perhaps, his anger that things have turned out the way they have. Without emotional supports from the adults around him—his grandparents, me, his uncle—I could imagine him becoming depressed, acting up, and potentially getting into trouble with the law, or being at risk for drug abuse. We can't live in the future, but by anticipating these dangers, we hope they may be prevented. That may be the most that we can do.

LOOKING BACK

Partially successful cases like this one are a familiar experience to anyone who has ever worked with troubled families. What this case has in common with many of them is the overwhelming impact of environment. For many of the families that are seen in clinic or agency settings, the difficulty lies not with motivation or ability to learn skills, but the multiple problems that seem to constantly badger the family—unemployment, poverty, illness—that keep the family in a crisis mode, and like this family, make it difficult to maintain a positive momentum. Even with all the family work and residential treatment available, these environmental forces may still drag them down. Ideally, through therapy they will have fewer internal distractions and acquire greater family resources to help them weather these emotional storms better.

What this case also illustrates is that all clinical work doesn't turn out smoothly, that with the best of intentions and skills, treatment can become derailed. Good clinical work is pragmatic: New approaches have to be tried, and often a combination of services need to be included, until the right fit is found. This case also demonstrates the circularity of the work, the way one path eventually connects to others. Therapy, for example, could have started with the family and moved toward individual work with Billy, or started with the marriage, if the couple would have permitted it, and then tied into Billy's concerns. The initial focus could have been on the school, helping them to better accommodate his needs or carrying their more structured approaches into the home. The starting point is in a sense arbitrary, merely an entrance in the larger system and system change.

Billy's story also illustrates the boundaries and limitations of each of the systems and institutions—the family's reluctance to change its way of parenting; the school's own goals, needs, and inability to control Billy's behavior; my own scheduling limitations in seeing Billy more often; the limited resources available for respite or home-based services; the limits of the community in responding with more expensive residential treatment only after all the other options had been tried. Such limits are part and parcel of every community's services, and are neither good nor bad, but obviously shape the decision-making process.

Finally, the story of Billy illustrates the resiliency of a child and family to survive trauma, and the inestimable effect that love and commitment can have. Without the family's ability to care for and see Billy for who he is an can be in the future, without some commitment on my part, perhaps, to stick with Billy and his family, rather than farm the family and their problems out along the way, it's easy to imagine Billy going from foster home to foster home, in and out of the hospital, increasingly locked in a downward cycle of negative behavior and self-fulfilling prophecies. Now his future, while still uncertain, is resting upon an increasingly larger base of past and present experiences that include people who only want the best that life can give him. In the life of a child, this often is the best we as adults can do.

Looking Within: Chapter 10 Exercises

1. If you haven't done it already, write down your own assumptions about problems in children. What is the major source of the problems—within, without? What is the role of development, of family, of the past? Where do the solutions lie? What is your primary role as the therapist?

2. What type of problems with children would you have the most difficulty with—acting-out 10-year-olds, sexually abused children, hyperactive or aggressive children, children who have suffered a loss—not only in terms of your skill, but your own emotional response? How are you to handle such cases and emotions—avoiding them by farming them out, becoming controlling, minimizing the problems, becoming overwhelmed and passive, overidentifying with the child?

3. If there was something from your childhood that you most regret, what would it be? What do you wish your parent or parents did more of for you? How do you wish your relationships with

your siblings were different when you were a child? What part of this has had an impact on your work with children now? How?

4. What skills do you most need to develop in working with children—play therapy, art therapy, psychological testing, work with younger children or older ones, integrating children in the family process? How could you learn those skills?

[11]

"See How She Treats Me!"
THE PARENT–ADOLESCENT STRUGGLE

"So, how was your week?"

Ms. Harris, a slight woman with graying blond hair and drooping shoulders, takes a quick glance at her 15-year-old daughter, Ellen. Although Ellen is slumped in the corner of the couch, it's easy to see that she's several inches taller and about 20 pounds heavier than her mother. Her head is turned away, and she's staring absently at the lamp.

"Okay, I guess," says Ms. Harris. She sounds tentative and glances again at Ellen. Ellen, still looking at the lamp, just breathes heavily.

"Actually, we did fine until I tried to get Ellen to clean up her room."

"I *did* clean my room!" snaps Ellen, whirling around to face her accuser. "*You* just didn't think it was good enough!" She is glaring.

"You left all those clothes all over the floor, after I asked you nicely to pick them up." Ms. Harris sounds almost angry, but she's holding back, being careful.

"I said I was going to wear them, didn't I?"

"Yes, but—"

"And then *you* wouldn't let me talk on the phone!"

"I asked you if you could call back later because I was expecting a call from Louis." Ms. Harris sounds a bit firmer this time.

"I told you I was almost done!"

The mother turns to the therapist. "And do you know what she did? I asked her again nicely to hurry up, and then she had a fit, ripped the phone right out of the wall, and threw it down on the floor!" She seems mad, but suddenly her lower lip is pouting out, and then she collapses into quiet tears. "I don't know why she needs to do things like that. I didn't raise her that way."

"Oh, you're pathetic!" sneers Ellen.

Welcome to the world of adolescence. Here in Ellen we see perhaps a larger version of what Billy potentially could become, and in some ways these families are similar. Just as Billy was dealing with the loss of his brother and parents, Ellen, and the two younger children, Marie, age 12, and Betsy, age seven, are all dealing with the death of Harry, their father and Ms. Harris's husband, of a heart attack a year and a half ago. Since then the family has struggled financially, with Ms. Harris working two jobs, and emotionally, as each of them tries to fill the hole in family, in their lives.

But it's Ellen who's the center of concern. She's the one who has gotten into fights at school, who's having rages, who tries to boss around her younger sisters and hits them when they don't do what she wants. She demands and challenges her mother, and feels entitled. Ms. Harris, in many ways like Billy's grandmother, makes feeble efforts to assert control but, more often than not, caves in. Here at the third session it's clear that both Ms. Harris and Ellen have some major changes to make if both are to survive this adolescence.

MOVING UP

But there are also significant differences between Billy and Ellen simply because of the differences in age. As we move up the developmental ladder from children to adolescents, there are dramatic shifts in the therapy process. Here's a quick list of some of the obvious ones:

• *The stakes are higher.* While an elementary school-age child like Billy may get suspended from school, or tear up his room when he is angry, teenagers like Ellen won't have much trouble taking drugs, shoplifting, getting pregnant, running away, or engaging in seriously dangerous activities that could have long-term consequences on their future.

• *Different parenting skills are needed.* Ms. Williams, under the worst conditions, could, with a little bit of help, always pick Billy up and put him in his room for time-out. Ms. Harris can't do that with Ellen. Parenting a teen requires an entirely different skill set—having a greater sensitivity for personal boundaries and a greater reliance on compromise and negotiation; the ability to know what battles to pick and which ones to let go; the ability to recognize the power struggles and not fuel them, to balance limit setting with nurturance. Many parents lack these skills or have trouble making the leap. They feel frustrated when what used to work no longer does or can.

• *Others outside the family have increasing influence.* Younger children are most affected by their home and school environments, environments created by adults who are in charge. Ellen, however, is not only reacting to her mother, or even internally to the loss of her father, but, like other teens, also to the wider circle of friends who pull her in various directions as she struggles to define for herself who she is. She is sensitive to how and what they think about her, and worries about how she fits in. These are the other voices that she hears in counterpoint to those of her mother.

• *Parents often under- or overreact.* Recognizing your waning influence, the risks intertwined within their decisions, the sense that the time you have to affect your child's life is quickly running out can intensify a parent's reaction. Some, in fear and panic, overreact and overcontrol— threatening, demanding, pushing their child—to be more responsible, to stay away from trouble, or, better yet, to not grow up at all. Others, swinging too far the other way, feel that it is too late to turn things around, and allow their child to have full rein over them and to make his or her own decisions. Such parents have essentially given up.

But what drives these over- and underreactions are the parents' memories of their own adolescence—a distorted still-life, perhaps, filled with the painful throb of past mistakes, ongoing regret over roads not taken, an aching awareness that they and their parents failed in important ways. Such memories push parents to try to stop history from repeating itself with their own children.

• *Therapists' reactions can be more intense.* It's not only the parents who are sensitive to the risks and dynamics of adolescence; so too are therapists. When an adolescent is referred for therapy by the court— the "one last chance" before being sent off to a correction center—it's the therapist, as well as the teenager, who's under the gun. When a therapist sees destructive family dynamics souring the child's life, but faces parents too overwhelmed or impotent to change them, when a therapist wants the best for adolescent but feels stifled by bureaucracy or limited community resources, the therapist, too, can feel that time is running out. He or she starts to believe that it is necessary to work hard and fast in order to avert dire consequences, or the therapist decides, like the parents, like the community, that it isn't going to matter and stops trying.

• *The adolescent has more opportunity to fill a surrogate role.* The elementary school-age child can, of course, learn to copy and fill roles in the family. We could imagine that if Billy had stayed with his mother, for example, he would, even at his young age, absorb and act out more and more the boyfriend's control or violence, or would step in to support her emotionally.

But as the adolescent moves closer to adulthood the pull to fill such roles becomes even stronger. Here we see the oldest son working full- or part-time to help support the rest of the family and giving the mother advice when she asks or even doesn't ask for it; the 16-year-old daughter who watches the kids and makes dinner while Dad is working late; or, as with Ellen, a 15-year-old who feels, as the father did perhaps, not only that she has some responsibility to direct her younger sisters, but also that her mother will do what she wants her to do without objection.

• *The adolescent can be more verbal.* One of the main differences between child therapy and adolescent therapy is the capacity of adolescents to do more "talk" therapy, rather than symbolically express themselves through play. The adolescents' vocabulary and comprehension are greater, and their world is more complex. Unlike the elementary school child, for example, whose sense of right and wrong is governed by whether or not someone punishes you, the teens are slowly developing the ability to think abstractly. Their notions of personal values, ethics, and morality are emerging and now can be asked about and discussed directly.

• *Confidentiality is more vital.* While confidentiality certainly exists between young children and therapists, it is flexible—because the children rely so exclusively upon their parents to help them negotiate through the world, the parents need as much information as possible in order to help the child. As children become older, begin to both separate from the parents and see themselves as more independent, they no longer need to nor want to rely as much on their parents to help them solve problems. The boundaries between them and their parents are more firm; they can now begin to help themselves, making confidentiality more absolute and important. As the therapist you need to work harder to both build trust and assure the adolescent that his or her confidence will be respected.

Even though child and adolescent work are clearly different, the shift from one to the other varies from family to family. There are many 14- or 15-year-olds who would rather paint than talk, just are there some 10-year-olds who wouldn't dare play a game or touch a toy. There are adolescents who, due to intellectual or physical handicaps or limitations, are developmentally delayed and may not only play more and talk less, but may need to be managed by their parents as if they were younger. While some teens can work well in the solitude of individual therapy, many others are intimidated by this intimacy, and do best in the familiar interaction of family therapy where they can bounce off parents and siblings.

The way to find out how "adolescent" an adolescent is to *ask*—about the teen's and the family's expectations, to *do*—to talk with the adolescent alone, together with the parents, to offer to play cards and see what happens, and most of all to *listen and watch*. What helps the adolescent open up? What stimulates the most energy? What seems to have the most impact? By the end of that first session you should have a pretty good idea of just where the adolescent sits on the developmental continuum and how you can best join with him or her.

FALLING APART

Of course, there are all those families that you'll never see, the ones who manage to survive the trials and tribulations of adolescence not only intact, but relatively smoothly. Why do some families struggle more than others?

As suggested earlier, some parents of teens simply reach the limits of their own parenting skills and knowledge. They can't make the shift from physical-authoritarian management to a verbal-negotiating one. The father who threatens to spank his six-foot-two son if he doesn't cut the grass by Friday is setting himself up to fail. But if that's all the father knows, if threatening physical punishment sums up his entire repertoire of skills, his influence over his child has effectively ended.

Some teens have similar struggles with their own skills and transitions. Their problem-solving or decision-making skills may be weak; they may have limited social skills; the transition from elementary to middle school, middle school to high school feels overwhelming. They have trouble shifting into adolescence and get stuck. Even though they are separating from their parents, they have a hard time crossing over and finding a place for themselves in the often competitive but potentially supportive world of peers. They are caught between these two worlds—of childhood and adolescence, of home and peers—and in neither. These teens often feel lost, and are filled with loneliness and isolation.

Adding fuel to these struggles are the ups and downs of normal physiological changes. The spiking of hormones leads to the spiking of emotions. Parents of 13-year-olds complain about the rapid shifts from explosive anger to explosive tears, to moodiness and withdrawal, and some parents weather this better than others. If a teen has low self-esteem or poor coping skills, he or she may not be able to verbalize feelings and strikes out instead; rather than seeking others who can provide help, a teen may hold in his or her feelings and questions and get depressed; rather than finding healthy ways of relieving the pressure and stress, such as sports or creative arts, another teen may turn to drugs, sex, or acting out.

Many parents invariably will blame their child's misbehavior on friends—it's that the group of lowlifes that he sees at school, it's those girls up the street who do anything they want, that crowd on the corner who are putting ideas in his head, leading her astray. And they may be. But what's wrong with this explanation is that it implies that if you eliminate the friends—move, place the child under house arrest, enforce a strict curfew—the child will be cured.

Maybe, but often not for long. Somehow the child manages to find another group of scruffy characters in the new neighborhood or drifts back to the group once the curfew is eased. The problem usually has less to do with the friends and more to do with the reflection of him- or herself that the teenager sees in them. Separating friends is only half the solution. The other half is improving the child's self-esteem. The teen needs help learning how to be more assertive, how to improve social skills, how to find and use healthy supports within the family and with new friends.[1]

When an adolescent, like Ellen, takes on an inappropriate role within the family system, both the parents' ability to manage the child

[1]For an interesting, evidence-based, family-therapy approach to dealing with the influence of peer groups see Scott Henggeler et al., *Multisystemic Treatment of Antisocial Behavior in Children and Adolescents*, Guilford Press, 1998.

and the child's abilities to cope are stressed. By replacing her father's role in the family, Ellen, at 15, is not only filled with a sense of over-responsibility but also entitlement and power. Her "top dog" position in the family, coupled with her mother's weak parenting skills, locks the dysfunctional system in place.

Similarly, the child who has been the scapegoat and a vicarious outlet for a parent's anger or the "good child" who secures his or her place only by complementing the scapegoat's role can each over time become more and more entrenched in their roles and extreme in their behaviors. The scapegoat's behavior, once tolerable, now escalates and comes to the attention of the community, while the good child is more set on showing just how good he or she can be.

Running underneath all these adolescent potholes of skills, stress, and roles are the parent's own history and the power of this history to repeat itself. Sometimes these are genetically based—the son whose father has a history of bipolar illness finds himself sliding into bouts of severe depression or the mother with ADHD finds that her son has similar problems with inattention, impulsivity, and hyperactivity. Oftentimes, however, it's the combination of role modeling, family dynamics, and environmental forces that work together to repeat the past mistakes from one generation to the next: The mother who was pregnant at 14, finds, in spite of her constant warnings, that her daughter is pregnant at 15; the father who never went beyond the ninth grade finds himself arguing with his son who wants to quit school and work at a gas station; the mother who married an alcoholic and abuser painfully watches her own daughter endure the same fate.

What drives the replaying of these scripts is not only or even necessarily the replaying of the content, but the recycling of the underlying family and environmental dynamics. While the mother harangues her 15-year-old daughter to be careful around the boys she associates with, she isn't aware that it's as much the haranguing itself and the subsequent rift in their relationship that propels the daughter into pregnancy, just as her own mother's haranguing did to her. The son who feels that what was good for his father should be good enough for him finds his father's arguments to stay in school hypocritical and dismisses them. The daughter who saw her mother abused by her father not only expects men to act this way and associates intimacy with violence, but unconsciously copies the victim role that her mother modeled.

Seeing this replication of your life in the life of your child is both painful and powerful, and often pushes the parents into counseling. It's also part of what creates the ambivalence and reluctance that such parents come to display. To look beyond their panic forces the parents to look not only at the forces affecting their child and family, but also, painfully, at the forces shaping their own past.

To talk about the life options open to a teenager and power of history to repeat itself is to talk about the fundamental challenge of adolescence, namely, leaving home and setting a course for adulthood. Every family creates its own emotional climate, its own escape hatches, its own ultimatums that let the adolescent know how, when, and in what direction to leave. Some seem hopelessly trapped within the narrow choices they have; others work so hard not to become their parent that they don't figure out how to become themselves; and some, through the helping hand of another adult in their life, find a way to step outside the environmental and family patterns to become someone different.

What about your own experience? If you look back on your own time of leaving home, your reactions to your parents' past, your relationships with other adults outside your family, what is the moral of the story of your own adolescence? What behaviors did you want to emulate, what was that emotional bottom line that you reached in your relationship with your parents that told you it was time to leave? What mistakes of theirs did you or they want you most to avoid? By being aware of your own personal triggers, your own unfinished business, you can better separate your clinical judgment from your personal reactions when working with parents and teens.

THERAPEUTIC GOALS: THE BIG PICTURE

Skill assessment and education are often good starting points for helping parents of teens. Framing problems as ones of skill is often less threatening to parents, and concrete suggestions can increase their own sense of power and control. Provide them with information about adolescent development—for example, needs for privacy, adolescents' sensitivity to hypocrisy, the testing of limits, even something about brain development and limited abstract thinking—to help normalize the behaviors that seem to aggravate them so much. Coaching them on how to detect the power struggles and stop them, how to raise sensitive topics, on understanding and using the power of positive feedback, on giving the child permission to talk about his or her anger or sadness, on knowing when to lay down the law, or how to achieve a united front are always invaluable bits of information that most parents welcome once they've had the opportunity to tell their story and express their own opinions and concerns. In many cases this all that is needed to stop the dysfunctional patterns.

Other times, of course, this isn't enough. They may know the information or you provide the information but they struggle to carry it out. The parents fail to take a united stand; they don't emphatically say to Tyrone that he can't go out; they complain, but don't go down to the school and talk to the teacher to find out why Helen is failing. Here we're back to problems within the hierarchy, perhaps within the marital relationship, among the family roles, or unresolved issues from the parents' past. We may be creating and missing seeing a parallel process in action in which the parents are responding to our seeming direction with the same resistance with which the adolescent responds to theirs. We're once again falling back to the basics—clarifying expectations, looking for what's missing, moving toward anxiety, following the process and blocking the dysfunctional patterns in the room and in the home, looking for the problems that might underlie the poor solutions that the presenting problems really are.

When it's clear to you that problems stem from the adolescent's inappropriate role and hierarchy within the family system, realigning the system is the obvious goal. In the session process you point out when the adolescent isn't acting like an adolescent, but an adult. You challenge the parents to set limits, to act as parents rather than peers. You give the parents permission to assert their power (though not be abusive) that you as therapist, the courts, the schools will all support. They need to know that teenagers, like Ellen, shouldn't be out of control or too much in control, and can learn to be responsible and appropriate. They need to understand that the bottom line is that the adolescent, because of his or her age, can't win, and that the community is on the parents' side.

This message is particularly valuable for single parents who feel overrun by all-too-powerful teenagers. Your saying this doesn't make it happen—the parents still have to confront their own anxiety about changing roles and learning new skills—but your challenge and support gives them a vote of confidence. The clinician, or more often the courts, serves, in fact, as the second parent, forming a united front to the child, which becomes the starting point for realignment.

But creating a workable structure is only half a solution. Parents need to provide positive attention and nurturing in order to give adolescents something to move toward, not only away from. Nurture and control go hand in hand. Often a parent, like Ms. Harris, feels comfortable with nurturing but struggles setting limits; for other parents the opposite is the case. In two-parent families, it's easy for the parents to polarize, with one's firm limits serving as a counter to the other parent's seeming softness and leniency. The united front collapses, and the teen splits and tries to maneuver through the cracks. Balance is necessary, a combination of clear and age-appropriate boundaries with love and attention, respect and appreciation. In embattled families, often the best place to start regaining control is to help parents to be more respectful and appreciative.

One of the most useful stances parents, especially of teenagers, can take is not personalizing their child's behavior or verbal attacks, that is, realizing that it is not about them, but rather a reflection of the child's own internal struggle. When the teen gets enraged, for example, it's helpful for the parents to see this as the teen's solution, albeit it a poor one, of dealing with some other emotions swirling within. By seeing the outburst or acting out as a sign that the teen is having a hard time rather than a preemptive malicious attack on the parents, the parents are better able to step back from the conflict, and can even show some compassion for the teen's struggle. In the moment the parents can be coached to do best by doing little—listening, reflecting back the teen's feelings—and avoiding the temptation to get angry themselves and defend their position. Such a counterattack only fuels the teen's emotions, rather than calming and changing the emotional climate.

But this can be difficult, especially for parents who were never nurtured themselves. They've learned to think of parenting as yelling, threatening, or slapping across the face or behind when a child gets out of hand. They worry that not counterattacking is letting the kid walk all over them, allowing him or her to be disrespectful of them, or teaching him that there are no limits. The parents need to be reassured that they can always restate and reset limits after the storm is over, even set limits at the time if necessary (e.g., call the police if the teen gets too aggressive). They need to constantly reassured that they do have the power, but can be most effective if they can avoid the power struggle.[2]

---

[2]An excellent guide for parents on understanding the world of adolescents and adopting these attitudes is found in Michael Bradley, *Yes, Your Teen is Crazy*, Harbor Press, 2003.

The way to best convey this attitude is not just to tell the parents to do it, but to model it—toward the adolescent (for example, nurture Mary by saying "Your teacher told me that you have been doing wonderfully the past week at school" or by remaining calm when Mary gets upset and begins to complain) and the parents ("From what you've told me about your father, Rochelle, it sounds like you did the very best you could for you and your sister—it must have been really tough for you," or listen sympathetically when the parent voices her frustration) in the session. The starting goal for any treatment plan is empowering parents to be parents. To do that you usually need to treat them the way they need to treat the adolescent.

While my personal style is to work as much as possible either coaching the parents on specific skills and stances, or doing family therapy with parents and teens to improve communication and negotiate problems, supportive individual therapy is a logical option for the teenager who's depressed, overwhelmed, or has poor self-esteem, and is struggling with the trials of adolescence. In chaotic or violent homes, giving the adolescent an opportunity to talk to an empathic adult, an ideal parent, not only can be a refuge but also a powerful corrective emotional experience. The teen learns that it can be safe to express yourself and take the risk of intimacy, that you can separate yourself from the craziness around you, that adults and the adult world are more varied and complex than the one-dimensional impressions they have understandably formed.

For adolescents who cope through self-abuse—cutting, eating disorders, addictions—individual therapy can help them learn the terrain of their emotional life. You can aid them in putting words to the thoughts and emotions that lie beneath the behaviors and teach them how to express them assertively. They can recognize the environmental and social triggers for the abuse, experiment with specific behavioral ways of breaking the cycle, and learn healthier, more appropriate means of coping.[3]

In most cases a combination of approaches is the most effective. Parents can be given guidelines on new and specific behavioral changes that they can begin to make in the home in order to avoid power struggles, break the dysfunctional patterns, and provide support. Individual therapy with teens can focus on helping them define their internal world and cho-

---

[3]There are a number of excellent specific texts and workbooks for clients who engage in various forms of self-abuse. One of the best overall books is Dusty Miller, *Women Who Hurt Themselves*, Basic Books, 1995.

reographing in advance their upcoming discussion with parents in family therapy about their needs or their appropriate, assertive voicing of complaints. Family therapy can be the forum for learning communication skills, problem solving, demonstrating nurturing skills to parents, drawing out the hidden sides of everyone's role, or clarifying the intention behind the behavior. An adolescent group, if available, can provide further opportunities for the development of social skills in a safe environment and can help reduce isolation. The confrontation by peers can have a far greater impact than such confrontation by a therapist, and accelerate change.

Whatever way you choose to support a teen, be alert to the dangers of usurping the parents' role. For parents who blame the child, who are passive, frustrated, or tired of trying to handle problems, stepping back and letting the clinician step in becomes all too easy. For the adolescent who feels misunderstood, resentful, and hungry for intimacy with an adult, a deep dependency upon the therapist becomes a real possibility. This doesn't mean that you should never take this approach; sometimes it is the best course to take. However, the clinician needs to make a deliberate clinical choice and be clear about his or her own commitment to the teenager.

Finally, when the forces of the parents' past are being replicated in the life of the adolescent, the starting point for assessment and treatment planning begins with the parents' own ability to see and understand how they have helped create the dynamics that have enabled the replication to happen. Following in one's footsteps is chalked up by some parents to fate or genetics—"My cousin had a boy just like Simon who wouldn't listen and he eventually got in big trouble with the wrong crowd"—as a given over which they have little control.

Others who see the shadow of their own lives mirrored in their child find it too painful and retreat into minimization and denial. What the adolescent is doing—shoplifting but not breaking into houses, dating older men but not pregnant at 13—is different enough or doesn't seem quite so bad to them as their own past; the problem, they decide, isn't with them, but only with the child or with the influence of friends. For still others this replication of history is all too apparent, but only creates enormous guilt and panic and little else; the forces that create the problem or how to change it are outside their awareness.

Your focus certainly doesn't need to be on the blame, but on helping the parents see that while their past is part of their own and their child's present, it's a present that can be changed. Parents need to know that they have to stay neither walled off by denial nor mired in guilt, but can increase their control and power by recognizing and changing the patterns and process that create and maintain the problems. The fact that the father is emotionally abandoning his son just as his own father physically abandoned him is less important than helping the father see his son succeed.

H. L. Mencken once said that most complex questions turn out to have a simple answer, but that's it's usually wrong. While it's simpler to talk of adolescent problems in terms of one source/one goal, in reality problems between parents and adolescents usually stem from several sources, all intersecting at one time—poor parenting and coping skills, an overwhelmed parent and adolescent, poor communication, and inappropriate roles and misalignments born out of the family's struggles with past losses, traumas, and environmental stress. Which you choose to focus upon the most will depend upon your theoretical frame, personality, and priorities.

If you are most comfortable thinking systemically, a lopsided hierarchy is what may stand out most in the first session. If you feel comfortable in the role of teacher, or come to see many of your families as warped by unrealistic expectations for teenagers and themselves, educating the parents on normal adolescent development and appropriate skills may naturally seem the best course. If you draw from a psychodynamic orientation, your work might entail seeing the adolescent individually to unravel defenses and increase insight. All of these are valid and can be effective; once again, there are many paths through the forest from which to choose.

But while your theory, comfort, and family expectations may be a starting point for your brainstorming, pragmatics and practicality need to be considered as well. If you work in an agency that has heavy caseloads, or find insurance limiting the length of treatment, you may need to think in terms of moving through problem and solution in layers, from the simplest and least interventionist to those more complex and long term.

For example, if a parent comes in complaining of a child like Ellen who is running the family, your structural understanding of the family would indicate that it is important to start by reinforcing the parental hierarchy. You might focus on helping the mother tighten up her parenting and set clearer limits as a first goal. If this works and the troublesome teen settles down and starts to get attention in more positive ways, therapy can be brief indeed. If, however, the mom has a hard time implementing the structure, or if the teen's depression over her peer relationships comes to the surface once her acting out stops, a shift can be made to family or individual work. These next layers of problems are only addressed if simpler solutions fail.

WALKING THE LINE: OPENING MOVES

If it seems that as a therapist you have to do a lot of juggling—between adolescents and parents, past and present, individual work and family work—you're right. Unlike treatment of younger children, working with adolescents requires walking a finer line, carefully balancing the adolescent's needs with those of the family.

The balancing you have to do reflects the awkwardness and precarious balance that both makes up adolescence and distinguishes it from childhood. Even though a child may be reluctant to come to therapy, his or her parents can make the child come, and usually rapport can be quickly established through play therapy. Even though the child may be under considerable personal stress, his or her sensitivity to and dependency upon the relationship with the parents and home environment makes it likely that the smallest of positive changes will ripple down and help the child. Even though the child may be severely acting out, he or she is unlikely to be under the gun of legal charges or decisions that can have lifelong consequences (e.g., abortion or adoption vs. becoming a teenage parent). Even though the parents of a seven-year-old may be worried about what the school says, there's a feeling that there is time to work it out.

This all changes with the adolescent. Instead of one or two adults and a child, there are one or two adults and another half adult, each side representing different cultures, with you as the bridge between them. Many therapists (especially those in their 20s and 30s, it seems) find it easy to identify with their adolescent clients and see them as the victims of rigid parents. Their efforts to get the parents to "loosen up" can quickly cause the parents to see the therapist (especially if he or she is younger than them) siding with their teen and not them. They quickly dismiss the therapist as being out of touch with the real world of parenting.

Your fate with the teen isn't much better. Because of your age, you are also seen by him or her as "one of them"—simply offering to play a game of checkers won't automatically win the teen over. While your ability to build rapport and ease anxiety in a child can often easily be done by his or her seeing you create a comfortable relationship with the parent, this same move with adolescents can backfire. If you seem to be too much on the side of parents, working too hard for their agenda, if there is any suspicion that confidentiality will be broken, the relationship never gets off the ground.

Your place in the middle between these generations means that your opening moves are extremely important. In order to build a foundation of rapport, you need to demonstrate to the teenager across from you that you are different from his or her parents. This doesn't mean that you have to know who's in Billboard's top ten, talk only in this year's street slang, do card tricks or break boards with karate chops, or have a tattoo the size of Montana on your forearm. It means that working with teens is like any other cross-cultural work: You need to show respect and a sincere interest in understanding the adolescent world. Ask questions ("What is school like for you?" "What is most difficult about being your age?" "What do you most wish you could do?") and demonstrate a patient willingness to listen.

But the parents are your customers as well. You can't leave them in the waiting room thumbing through old issues of *Time* magazine for a couple of months wondering what's going on in there and what they're paying for. Their place in the hierarchy of the family, their anxiety, and often their problems, including the behavior of their child, requires you to include them.

As with the younger child, part of your assessment is figuring out just how much time you need or want to spend with each family member, which problem (parent's or child's) has the higher priority, which treatment format (individual, couple, family) is the best approach. As with children, as one option closes—the adolescent thinks you're a jerk and never comes back—the others remain open. All is not lost.

Still, it's easy to wind up feeling like a bouncing ball if you're not careful, shuttling back and forth between the generations like a state-department diplomat. The way out of this is not to think in terms of being *between*, but *above*; your client isn't the adolescent, or the parent(s), or even the adolescent *and* the parent(s), but the family system.

Your role needs to be clear. Your job in those first few sessions is to build rapport with and trust on both sides, gather information, develop a therapeutic contract with the parent(s) and the adolescent regarding their goals. If possible, use your understanding of the family dynamics and the structural problems to link those goals together.

Kamesha, for example, is infuriated with her mother, who won't ever let her go out with her friends; her mother is furious with Kamesha because the only thing she seems to talk about is wanting to go out. You could help both of them see how they are having a power struggle and polarizing each other, as well as help Kamesha talk about how she would like to spend time with her mother, or better yet, explore whether her wanting to go out stems at least in part from the tension and criticism she feels when she's at home. You could help the mother talk about her own teenage experiences and how they may fuel her fears about her daughter going out, the way she feels rejected by Kamesha, or how her complaining may simply be her way of getting Kamesha to pay some attention to her. Rather than mediating how much time to spend with friends, your goals become helping mother and daughter become curious about the role of this issue in their lives, and encouraging them to find positive ways of communicating and spending time together.

Similarly, when Adam complains that his parents are always on his back, and his parents complain that Adam isn't doing his schoolwork and isn't conscientious like his older brother, the problem isn't schoolwork or criticism but helping Adam move out of a scapegoat role. The parents need to know that they can help Adam with school by first seeing him as different than his brother, while Adam can be challenged to get his parents off his back by finding other ways of gaining their attention and helping them see him for who he is.

Your job then is see what parent(s) and adolescent may not—their blind spots—and to offer a perspective that incorporates both sides of the problems. You need to say and show from the onset that you're not working for one or the other, but both. Successful adolescence is, after all, the ability to integrate into the family growing differences and needs.

While you're clear about what you'll do, you're also clear about what you won't do. Some of these limits are dictated by your theoretical model: No, you will not only do individual therapy with the teenager to fix him or her; yes, it is important that the father attend the sessions, or that the couple come in together to work on their communication and conflicts. Others are the legal and ethical limits of confidentiality: You will need to notify parents if there is suicidal or homicidal risk; you will need to contact protective services if abuse or neglect is suspected.

It's best to clarify these ethical and legal limits as soon as possible. In some settings this may be done for you by those handling intake. You need then to only follow up to see if the family understands or has questions. Some therapists define the rules of confidentiality matter-of-factly at the beginning of treatment. I tend to give the family members a two-page, simply written handout at the first appointment that includes information on contacting me in emergencies, failed appointment policy, payment of fees, a few statements about my style and approach, and a statement on confidentiality. I ask that they sign that they have read it and understand it, and make sure I follow up to see if they have any questions no later than the second appointment. I also discuss with them as soon as possible my desire to coordinate services with other professionals or agencies working with them and my need for appropriate releases of information.

However your choose to approach this, the key here is to be clear, informative, and matter-of-fact. Overemphasizing this can make some families anxious and suspicious even if they feel they have nothing to hide—they don't even know you, and you're already talking about how you may turn them in. While it can be tempting to avoid some of this awkwardness by putting off discussing confidentiality until the situation comes up, this always backfires. The family feels deceived and angry that you weren't up front and clear. By getting the limits of confidentiality on the table at the beginning, clients are able to decide for themselves how much and when to disclose.

In addition to defining your role, good beginnings require that you be careful to create symmetry and balance. Seeing the entire family at the start of the first session has the advantage of not only helping you see how they interact right away, but reduces the paranoia that family members have at being left out of the session. If there's a need to see the parent and teenager separately—to build rapport, to see what each is like apart form the other, to educate or discuss material inappropriate for the other (parents' or teens' sex lives, marital issues, details of what the teen may do outside the home)—that's fine as long as the time is balanced, and you are clear in your plan so that both sides have an overall sense of what's going on. The quickest way to build paranoia in a teenager or anxiety in a parent is to leave either one of them out in the waiting room for a few sessions with the magazines while the others are back in the office with you. Once you've finished your assessment and you have discussed and come to a consensus with everyone on the type of treatment format that will be used, the balance becomes less crucial.

ASSESSMENT: THE ADOLESCENT VARIATIONS

Because most families with teenagers enter therapy in a state of war, you need to move quickly to calm things by helping everyone have his or her say, by taking both sides and helping them see in the room how everyone bounces off of each other without even being aware of it. But once the dust has settled you need to gather the information you need to establish a treatment plan. The assessment of an adolescent and his or her family is not much different than any other family—you still want to see the patterns, define the problem, see what's missing, clarify the family's theory of the problem, and so on. However, the adolescent stage of development prompts some additional questions, especially those surrounding communication, problem solving, and rapport that you may want to ask yourself and/or the family members. Here's a quick checklist broken down by who's in the room:

Parent(s) and Adolescent

Who's missing from the session—father, mother, other siblings? Why? Important but absent members may potentially undermine the treatment.

Who's the most active? Often this reflects what happens at home; sometimes it merely shows who's the most motivated or anxious.

Who's got the problem; that is, who's the customer? Mother? Father? Court? School? There may be more than one, but you want at least one in the room.

What is the emotional climate in the room? Angry? Depressed? Anxious? The emotional climate is like taking the family's temperature. One of tasks for the first session may be to change the climate or uncover what can change it.

How does the adolescent respond to the parents, to you? Quiet? Argues back? Silently defiant? Again you're wondering how much this matches what happens at home (go ahead and ask) and whether it might be better to see the teen alone in order to built rapport and get a better perspective on what he or she is really like.

How well can the parents articulate their concerns? What the teen usually hears, of course, is the criticism, the parent on his or her back. Can you help the parents help their child to understand the *fear* and *worry* that underlie the parents' attitude?

Can the adolescent articulate a logical, rational counterargument? Adolescents are like novice lawyers, trying to argue their case with little experience and only the basic skills. Through the arguing, however, by trying to state their reasons and rationalizations aloud, they not only further develop the corners of their brains that handle abstract reasoning, they actually are forced to discover and define what they believe and think, all helpful life skills to have. Teens who complain or get angry about parental limits but little else need to learn to use their emotions as information about what they need or don't like and come up with a counteroffer.

Some teens all too quickly collapse under the weight of parental reasoning (teens who abuse themselves with cutting or eating disorders often do this), and tend to cope with the anxiety of conflict by being good— they switch and agree with the parents or backpedal from their own request. They need support in holding their ground. Let them know that their feelings are important, their position is reasonable, and help them articulate it. Coach the parents to back off and listen so that the teen feels safe enough to come out of the corner. Help them understand that what is at stake is not the details of the argument, but their teen finding his or her voice and learning to approach, rather than flee, from conflict. When they hear good, reasonable thinking coming their way, encourage the parents to allow themselves to be persuaded.

Can someone stop when things get out of control? Police don't count. Whether it's one of the parents who calls a halt to escalating arguments or an adolescent who stomps off and slams shut the door of his or her room, what's important is that someone is able to stay sane enough to realize when the process is getting out of control. Some families are unable to do this type of self-regulation, and the results are verbal abuse or even physical violence. If this begins to happen in your office, it's essential that you step in and stop it. If they can't be civil in the same room, separate them, and focus first on teaching them how to stop.

Are the parents presenting a united front or are they split? Splitting leads to teens working the parents against each other or their falling through the cracks.

Can the parents say positive things about the child? We are what we hear, and research says that we need a 3:1 ratio of positive to negative comments in order for us to be able to even hear the positives. In highly conflictual families, being aware of positives can be a stretch. Parents need to be coached and complimented themselves by you in order to change their ways.

How does the family respond to you? What are their expectations of counseling? Some parents are looking for an arbitrator, someone to straighten their teen out, or parenting advice; a few are actually looking for family therapy. Most teens are likely looking to get out of the room as quickly as possible; discovering that you are not just like their parents, that you have some understanding what life as a teenager is like is often a welcome relief.

The fact that teenagers and parents have different points of view is a given. What you don't want to reinforce by your inactivity, especially in the first session and especially with teens who can't hold their own ground, is an ongoing replication in the room of the dysfunctional dynamics. If the adolescent sees you sitting there watching him or her getting bashed on both sides by parents, his or her confidence in your ability to protect or even understand his or her point of view is severely handicapped.

Adolescent Alone

How well and willing is he or she to articulate his or her point of view? Some struggle because of developmental delays; some because they get anxious talking to adults; some because they don't want to be there and get passive-aggressive. You need to understand what might be going on and help the teen get his or her story out.

What is his or her theory about the problems in the home? How much self-awareness is present? How much blame, guilt? Again, in the theory lies the solution. Creating rapport, developing trust means understanding the teen's world and problems. While most teens see themselves, in varying degrees, as victims of the adult world, they also vary in their ability to step outside themselves and empathize with someone else's point of view (I know my parents are worried; I don't expect them to let me do whatever I want). Excessive blame makes it more difficult to move toward problem solving, while excessive guilt absorbs the energy that could be used for new behavioral changes.

How does he or she relate to siblings? What role does he or she take in the family system? Are siblings an emotional support or stress? The honor-society, football-quarterback older brother can be an impossible act to follow or a source of inspiration and support. The acting-out younger sister can be a pain in the neck or an additional source of worry and pressure. If you haven't seen the interaction among them in a total family session, you want to know about relationships with siblings. Teens who have a bond with their brothers and sisters are not only less stressed and less lonely, but potentially have in-house support for changes.

Does he or she have friends? Is he or she a leader or follower? How much do friends provide support? How strong and what type of influence and modeling do they provide? Most adolescents will tell you about their place in the peer hierarchy without any trouble. Of particular concern are the isolated adolescents who have few supports, no best friends. They have nothing to hold onto as they try to separate from parents and are at greater risk for depression, drug abuse.

Does he or she have a boyfriend or girlfriend? What is the quality of the relationship? How much is it a source of support or stress? Does the current one follow the same pattern as the intimate relationships before? How all-encompassing is the relationship—is there room for relationships with other friends? Is the relationship sexual? Is it responsible? Does it replicate the parent's history in some way, or the marital relationship? Basically, is the intimate relationship a positive or negative force in the teen's life? Is the teen in that relationship a better person than he or she seems at home, or is it more of the same?

Does he or she use drugs? What kind? How often? Is there an addiction that needs treatment before any further therapy should be undertaken? Just matter-of-factly asking about these drugs often, surprisingly, will give you information, especially if your tone is one of concern rather than criticism. Looking at family history (for example, Dad is an alcoholic) and risk for self-medication through drugs (social isolation, poor social skills, depression, hyperactivity, etc.) should raise your antenna and give you a context for talking to the teen about this: "You mentioned that your dad drinks a lot. How about you—how much do you drink?" [It's better to matter-of-factly assume the positive and get a denial than ask if he or she does drink.] "Do you worry that you could become a heavy drinker like him?"

Some teens will deny drug use at the beginning, but once they trust you, they will bring it up on their own. If an adolescent is addicted, use the therapy to get the adolescent into drug treatment, and keep in touch while in treatment. Don't expect, however, to do effective family therapy with an untreated addicted teen.

School—an arena of accomplishment and success or failure? Are educational goals realistic? Are relationships with teachers supportive or antagonistic? Are there any apparent intellectual, emotional barriers to success? How is classroom behavior? Is work completed? Does the he or she fit in with a group? Is he or she a loner? Adolescents have a home life, a school life, a street life. It doesn't take much, it seems, for some kids to give up on themselves as successful learners. Those with undiagnosed learning disabilities, ADHD, family struggles, emotional difficulties can come to view school as a place of failure and criticism, and their only friends are similarly burned-out types. The challenge is to help teens use school effectively, rather than just marking time until they can quit.

Does the teenager have dreams of the future? Are they realistic? Can he or she plan the steps leading to the goal? How are the goals shaped by the parents' expectations, other siblings, the parents' own history? This is a more sophisticated version of the childhood question, What do you want to be when you grow up? The 100-pounder who wants to become a pro wrestler needs help going from passion to practicality. The 17-year-old who sees no point to life needs your help to resolve grief, trauma, or depression. Having dreams of the future provide the escape hatch from the often powerless feelings of adolescence.

How does he or she relate to you? Open? Closed? Suspicious? Accommodating? Passive? Defiant? Anxious? What is the contrast between the content and process from the session together with the parents? Think again in terms of what is missing, emotional range. Not being treated like the parents is a good sign.

Does he or she understand confidentiality and its limits? Confidentiality is important but so is their understanding the limits, especially when working with depressed teens.

What would he or she most like to be different at home? This question is particularly important for in it is the therapeutic contract. By asking the question you are telling the adolescent that you are not just dealing with the parent's agenda, but also his or her own as well. You're saying that this is the place to work on and accomplish what he or she wants, and offering him or her a stake in the process. Your task, of course, is to link the goals of the adolescent and parent so that one creates the other, or so both can be worked on simultaneously.

Parent(s) Alone

How do they see their relationship with their child? How would they like it to be? These questions can shift the discussion from what is wrong inside the child to the interpersonal interaction. Asking what they would like is beginning to define their side of the therapeutic contract.

Can they clearly articulate the behavioral changes they most want to see? Most parents say they want their child to change his or her "attitude," too vague a goal. The parents need to be absolutely clear about what they are looking for, behaviorally and specifically, so the adolescent clearly knows what's expected.

What is their theory of the problems? Is it realistic, balanced? Do they see their own role? Is blame given to outside forces such as teachers, friends? Do they show empathy for their child? If everyone else is to blame, the parents are victims who feel that they can do nothing to fix the problems.

Is the adolescent the family scapegoat? What roles do the other children in the family play? Is there is a role for the adolescent to move toward? If Mary is the smart one, Tommy the athletic one, Jane the cute one, and Eric the popular one, there may be no role for Brian except to be the delinquent one or Claudia to be the depressed one. Often helping parents see how easy it is for them to lock on to narrowest slice of their children's abilities and personalities is enough to start to expand family roles.

Who is most involved with the adolescent? How enmeshed is the relationship? How appropriate? Who is more distant? Why? Dad may only show up to yell at Carlos to take out the garbage, but the grandfather is a steady presence. Mom may wind up complaining to 15-year-old Nadine about her menopause because she has trouble making friends on the job.

How is the marital relationship? How is the adolescent triangled in? How are conflicts resolved? Is the adolescent fulfilling a surrogate role? Is there addiction or other disability handicapping one of the parents and the marital relationship? Most of the traditional schools of family therapy say the marital relationship is the core of the family. If the marriage is strong, then the parents are united, the parental hierarchy is in place, and there's not the need to use the child as part of a triangle to drain off anxiety between the couple.

How empathic can the parent(s) be of the child? Some parents have forgotten what it was like to be an adolescent themselves, or, because their child has more materially than they did, they believe the child should happy. Similarly, some parents expect a 14-year-old to act as responsible as a 30-year-old, and stay in a continual state of frustration.

Are their goals for counseling realistic? If they think that they will drop their teen off for two sessions so you can sit down with him or her and "straighten out" the teen, they are going to be miffed when you ask them if they could to block out five o'clock on the next ten Tuesdays for family sessions. Find out what they expect.

Is the child re-creating the parent's history? How is this fueling the parent's response? What does the parent think the child most needs in order to be a success in life? Help the parents separate the past from the present, themselves from their children. Children represent new potential and a wide open future. If their adolescent represents a chance for the parents to correct all their past mistakes or to live their lives over, they are setting themselves up for struggle and disappointment.

How do the parents present differently alone with you versus with the teen or the rest of the family? What is the gap between your view and knowledge of the adolescent and their own? What do they need to most learn about their child? Parents can easily wind up showing only one side of themselves to their children, which deprives the children of broader role modeling and an understanding of what their parents really are like as people. Similarly, many parents are not able to see their own blind spots concerning their child and will need help expanding their view.

How do they relate to you? What role have they placed you in? Is there good rapport? If you're closer to their teenager's age than theirs, or if they're wary because you don't have any kids, you may have to work harder or differently to gain their trust.

Is there another parent or parental figure that you need to see? If Grandma really is the power in the family, you need to get her involved.

Who else do you need information from? Court? Schools? Do they understand confidentiality and its limits between you and them, between you and the adolescent? Make sure the adolescent gives consent for information, not just the parents.

Whole Family

Who's in charge? What's the comfortable problem? You can discover both of these answers by watching the process. Who represents the family—the father, mother? Who talks the most or for everyone else and tells you exactly what the problem is? Maybe the kids act up and the parents do nothing, causing you to wonder if this is what happens at home and is part of the problem. What problem or person does the family always return to, especially to break a silence or when you ask an anxiety-provoking question ("So what happens when you both have marital arguments?"). This problem, that person is what everyone is comfortable talking about. This is where the fingers point when less comfortable problems get raised at home.

How do the siblings interact? What roles do they play out? What are the coalitions and competitions? How are they joined or split between the parents? In large families the children may be broken up into camps—the boys with Dad, the girls with Mom; Kevin is Mom's favorite, Tina is Dad's. The family is split, the children have divided loyalties; through sibling rivalry the children may act out the marital tension.

What's the siblings' theory about the problems? What would they like to see changed? How do they see the adolescent differently than the parents? How do they perceive the marriage? When the children are not split into camps, they can often give a more balanced, reasonable view of the problem—"I think my parents are too tough on Ray, but he shouldn't get them mad by staying out late." This perspective gives you something to bounce off the family, such as, "Do you think what Amy says is true?" It gives you a good place to start.

How are conflicts resolved in the process of the session? How are the parents and the adolescent both different with the rest of the family than they are individually? Who backs down, who is the compromiser, who sides with the mother? Is there good discussion or are there threats and hysteria? You want to know how the process breaks down so you can help them change it.

If you notice that the family acts differently when they are all together than when they are not, you want to understand why. The differences may say something about the family culture, the way the children get attention, the impact of allies and divisions among the family members. Dad, for example, may sound strong and stern when talking together with his wife, but in the family session Mother joins with the rest of the kids in discounting him. Simply noticing the change aloud can help the family uncover the dynamics that propel them.

Are there additional family problems that are not being acknowledged? Do other family members have goals that would help break the dysfunctional patterns within the family? Although neither the parents nor the teenager have mentioned it, you discover in the family session that the youngest son has cerebral palsy or a cleft lip. Or maybe the four-year-old blurts out that Grandma went to jail last month. These are the problems beneath the presenting problems, family stressors that may be precipitating both the struggle the family is having and their coming in for counseling.

Do the parents see the session as valuable or irrelevant to their primary concerns? Back to expectations. Some parents wonder why you want to waste their time and money talking to the six-year-old twins when the problem is their 15-year-old. Others are surprised by what they learn from the mouths of the other family members, or come to see that the problem isn't just their teenager, but their parenting or the fact that Dad drinks a lot. The way to know what they think about it is to ask.

How do you feel dealing with so many people at one time? Not only may this give a sense of how the parents may feel much of time, but also how reasonable it may be for you to do whole family sessions.

Of course you will not have to ask all these questions—some may be obvious to you as you watch the family, some may be clear through the given background information, and some may not fit your own theory and you will substitute others instead. The point of the questions and the assessment, however, is to see how the lives of the family members overlap and stumble on each other, to find the places where functional interactions break down, to discover the ways coping mechanisms and inner and outer resources can be harnessed to solve the problems. They open the door to the treatment possibilities.

Looking Within: Chapter 11 Exercises

1. How comfortable are you with teenagers in general? Are there certain problems, ages, gender, or personalities that are emotionally more difficult for you to understand or work with? Why?

2. When you look back at your own adolescence, what was most difficult about it? What do you most regret about that time? How have those regrets possibly shaped your current life?

[12]

The Parent–Adolescent Struggle II

THE RETURN OF MS. HARRIS AND ELLEN

Ms. Harris had made the appointment at the suggestion of the school guidance counselor, who was concerned not only about Ellen's fighting and poor grades, but also her grief. During one interview with the counselor Ellen started talking about her father and seemed to the counselor to be depressed. As Ms. Harris related this during that first session with Ellen, Ms. Harris herself began to tear up and talk about how hard their father's death had been on the kids. Ellen looked away and said that the school counselor was making a big deal about nothing.

That entire first session was spent seeing mother and daughter together, gathering history and information. It was clear that Ms. Harris was overwhelmed by the changes that her husband's death had brought, both economically and emotionally. She spoke freely and painfully about the past year. Most all she talked about how worried she was about Ellen, and her own guilt that she was not doing a good enough job as a mother.

Throughout all this Ellen acted stoically. When she wasn't answering a question with a grunt, it was with a simple yes or no, and she usually contradicted what her mother had said. The only change that she said she wanted at home was for her mother not to complain so much, and let her do more of what she wanted ("All her friends could!"), especially taking her to the mall on Saturdays. She, however, did agree to come back with her mother.

The second session was split between Ms. Harris and Ellen, to see how each was different without the other, to gather more history from Ms. Harris about her marriage, to build some rapport with Ellen. Ms. Harris was seen first so that even if Ellen worried that the therapist and mother were talking about her, at least she wouldn't worry that the therapist was repeating what she'd just told him.

When Ms. Harris talked about her husband her ambivalence was apparent. Once again in that crumbled, teary posture she described her husband as 15 years her senior, a long-standing alcoholic, verbally abusive at times, demanding and controlling of her and the children. Ms. Harris had appeased him as much as possible, served as a buffer between him and children, swallowed her own anger, and adapted a codependent role. His sudden death knocked her off her feet. Although she had worked part-time before, she now was holding down two jobs.

While she had no trouble with the two younger girls, Ellen's behavior was compounding the stress; having never needed to take a strong role with the children, she now was struggling to reshape her role and image in their eyes. While things certainly weren't great when he was alive, now they seemed absolutely awful. What she felt most was that she had to learn to be strong for the children.

Ellen by herself continued to exude her tough air. No, she didn't think about her father that much; yes, things had changed a lot in the past year and a half; yes, school was boring; no, her mother wasn't doing a good job, in fact, she was pathetic the way she whined and complained and gave her a hard time about going out with her friends, but she was even more pathetic because she would eventually give in if Ellen pushed long enough. And Ellen was the one who had to look after her sisters all the time either because her mother was working or she was tired. She didn't mind doing it too much, but her mother sure didn't seem to appreciate it.

The therapist let her vent, empathized with her feeling that things were unfair and that she was taking on more than most other kids her age had to. She just shrugged, but seemed to relax. The therapist talked to her about confidentiality, about therapy as a place to make some of the changes that may be important to her.

One of the traps here, of course, is to be seduced by Ellen's apparent strength and insight, to do as the mother does and give her too much power, to ask her what she thinks the mother or her sisters need most. But that only reinforces her distorted role. Her concern should only be on what she needs; it's up to Ms. Harris to be responsible for the rest.

The third session with Ms. Harris and Ellen together, with which we opened, showed just how the interaction between them is played out. Here they were replicating in the office what happens at home. Even with the therapist's support, Ms. Harris had a difficult time acknowledging her anger and not caving into Ellen, and Ellen had a hard time not becoming angry and scolding her mother. The third session ended with the therapist talking individually to the mother about specific parenting skills.

DOING WHAT WHEN

So what do we have here? As we saw with Billy, we have another parent who is having trouble setting limits. Ms. Harris not only is having to shift gears from parenting a younger child to a teenager, but is having to change roles within the family structure, from an ally and nurturer of the children to nurturer *and* disciplinarian. Ellen, due to her age, personality, and probably past patterns of relationship to her father and mother, has stepped into the father's role, and, together with her mother, is quickly replicating the marriage, complete with verbal abuse. The heightened sense of power that she has, along with her overresponsibility and concern for her sisters is enough to keep her in the role; what she's missing is any closeness with her mother or the opportunity to simply focus on her own life. Struggling with Ellen is a variation of her struggle with her husband and familiar ground for the mother, less anxiety-provoking than making the changes in her role that she needs to make, especially since she is already so overloaded.

So mother and daughter complement and interlock. Ellen takes charge because her mother doesn't, her mother doesn't because Ellen does. Ellen doesn't get sad, she (like her father did) gets angry, tough, and controlling. Ms. Harris doesn't get tough, she gets sad and helpless. Both, pulled by familiarity and pushed by complementarity, stay within their own comfortable emotion and behaviors. The anxiety, what's missing, the need for each is the same—to expand their emotional range and move toward the underside of what they each cannot now feel, rather than depending upon the other to play it out.

What this raises is the question of timing—deciding when it's best to do what, figuring out the sequence of steps needed to learn new skills and solve problems. Issues of timing run alongside the issue of depth (moving from the least to the more intrusive), alongside questions of priorities determined by the hierarchy of needs (e.g., getting the family on food stamps or helping Johnny get back in school before working on "growth" issues like understanding why you feel annoyed when your husband asks what's for dinner). The question of timing is knowing when to approach a topic or task in terms of the family's emotional readiness and foundation of skills. What does the family need to do first before they will be psychologically ready to do more?

If, according to your theory, you believe that it's unresolved grief as much as anything else that is driving the emotional reactions and roles in this family, then the question and the solution lies in determining how to facilitate the grief reaction. Like Billy, it's clear that Ellen isn't comfortable approaching the topic or feelings head on, and Ms. Harris, for all her sadness, can only go so far—after a year she is still too quickly immobilized by these sad emotions that only trigger Ellen's complementary anger. Like the parents of other overresponsible children and adolescents, Ms. Harris may need to step up before Ellen can step down. Before we can help Ellen more openly grieve we may have to help Ms. Harris get strong. To push Ellen to give up her toughness and look at her sadness while she sees her mother still wallowing and incapacitated may be too difficult for her.

One way of increasing individual power is to help clients become more aware of and able to express their anger. As part of the normal grief process, we can suspect that the Harris family members feel varying amounts of anger over the father letting them down. Anger is an important emotion because it is the beginning of boundary setting (knowing what you don't like), and physiologically is an antidote to energy-draining depression. But expecting Ms. Harris to quickly tap her anger as a way of feeling stronger may be too threatening and anxiety-provoking for someone who has spent most of her life suppressing such strong feelings. She may need to approach her anxiety more gradually, to take behavioral risks that increase her self-confidence and self-esteem before she feels capable of handling her own anger and feels entitled to express it.

This way of thinking, this mapping out of sequences and deciding which holes to move toward first can seem complex but isn't. All it involves is approaching a pocket of anxiety and seeing where the resistance most arises. Ms. Harris's own history with her husband, her difficulty in mobilizing her anger within the session with Ellen, gave the therapist immediate information and feedback about what may or may not work. If the mother had been able to stand firm to Ellen's demands, or if Ellen was able even in individual sessions to let down her guard and approach some of her feelings about her father, these would be clues that more direct routes could be taken. But they didn't happen, and to push either person too hard, so early toward what they most fear runs of risk of them shutting down or leaving treatment all together.

What we still don't know, however, is just how pervasive the grief is throughout the family, how entrenched both Ms. Harris and Ellen are in their roles, and the part the other girls play in maintaining the system. This is a good time to see the other children in a whole family session.

BRINGING IN THE REST OF THE TROOPS

They march in a single file down the hall, Ellen leading the way, followed by Betsy, skipping and jumping, then Marie, slouching, watching her feet, and finally Ms. Harris, once again bedraggled and frail looking. Ms. Harris dumps herself onto a couch alongside Betsy; Ellen sits by herself on the other one; Marie sits in the chair in-between.

"So, did your mom talk to you both about coming here today?"

Both Betsy and Marie nod.

"Momma, can I go over there and play?" asks eight-year-old Betsy.

Before Ms. Harris has a chance to say something, Ellen pipes up, "You need to stay here with us."

"Ms. Harris, I think Ellen spoke for you. Do you want Betsy to stay here next to you?"

"Sure, I guess. Honey, just sit here for a few minutes." Ms. Harris pulls Betsy close beside her.

"Your mom and Ellen and I have been talking in the past couple of weeks about all the changes that have been going on in your family. It sure sounds a lot has happened in the past year since your dad died."

"My Momma has to work a lot," says Betsy with a sigh, "and Ellen is always bossing us around."

"I do not!" snaps Ellen. "You're the one who's always bugging me, always running to Momma, always getting your way!"

"But you hit me!" And she lifts up the edge of her shorts and points to a faint black and blue mark.

"Girls, girls, please don't start," says Ms. Harris as she limply waves her hand toward both of them.

"Is this what happens at home, Marie?"

"All the time." She sounds bored.

"What do you do when they get into it?"

"Go to my room. Wait till they are finished."

"How are you and Ellen doing?"

"Okay. She tries to boss me around sometimes, but I just don't pay attention to her."

What's happened so far? We see Ellen assuming a parental role, both in the session process and at home, with little resistance from her mother. We could guess that Ms. Harris is closest to Betsy (she identifies with Betsy's helplessness?), is openly favored by her, and Ellen knows it, only increasing the gap between her and her mother, and her retaliation against Betsy. She and Ellen do battle where Ms. Harris does not. And Marie, just as she is seated in the room, is somewhere in between, the neutral middleman, who ducks for cover when conflict breaks out.

What we still need to know is how the family has crystallized around the father's death. After spending some time building rapport with Marie and Betsy, and finding out about their relationship with each other and their mother, this is where the focus turns:

"Betsy, it sounds like you are very close to your mom. How about your dad, were you close to him?" the therapist asks gently.

"Well, sort of, I guess. He would take me to the park sometimes, and sometimes I would sit on his lap when we were watching television."

"How did you feel when he died?"

"I was real sad, especially when I went to the funeral. Everybody was crying. . . . I stayed close to Momma. . . . "

Out of the corner of his eye the therapist sees that Marie is beginning to tear up.

"Marie," says the therapist softly, "what's wrong?"

Marie starts to cry harder.

"She feels sad," says Betsy.

"Are you thinking about your dad?"

Marie nods.

Ellen turns away and starts to get restless. "How about you Ellen, how are you feeling?"

Ellen ignores the question.

"Ms. Harris, how are you doing?"

"I know this is hard on the girls," she responds. "I don't bring this up at home or try and let them see me get upset."

"Sometimes Momma cries," says Betsy.

"And how to do you feel when you see her that way?"

"Bad, sad."

"Who do you all think misses your dad the most?"

Ellen can't handle this anymore. "This is a bunch of shit." She suddenly stands up and walks out of the office.

Grief gone underground. Ms. Harris tries to hold it within, crying secretly, hoping no one will see, making the grief itself a family secret. Marie, too, it turns out, does a lot of her own crying and missing of her father, but like the fights, steals off to her room. Betsy, like the little boy in *The Emperor's New Clothes*, isn't afraid to say what she sees and takes the junior caretaker role, the emotional backup when any sadness breaks out; like her mother she plays out the softer side of Ellen's anger and control. And Ellen, with everyone else morose and collapsing, is boxed in with her anger. Overwhelmed with such strong feelings from everyone in the family, she has no choice but, like her dad perhaps, to leave.

So our hypothesis is checked out. The grief is pervasive in the family, Betsy has stepped in as her mother's support and surrogate to re-create the marital tension; Marie, in many ways like her mother, is most comfortable stepping aside; and Ellen clearly is not able to tackle her own feelings of grief until the family gives her some room and helps her find a place. Ms. Harris needs to become the hub of the wheel, not to re-create her husband's role, but to include it within the new reality of her life as a single parent. Unless she can do that the children will continue in their adaptive styles, with Ellen winding up out of the family, Betsy eventually taking care of her mother, and Marie sitting alone, depressed, in her room.

One of the biggest traps with this family, as it was with Billy's grandmother, is the therapist stepping in and replacing the father as family head. This dynamic can most easily be recognized not only by mentally considering the likely replacement role in advance, but by emotionally feeling the pull to do so in the session process. Ms. Harris could reflexively look to the therapist for leadership, Betsy and Marie would find someone besides their mother to rely upon, and Ellen, although she may balk initially at having her position threatened, might be happy turning things over to this seemingly more capable adult, especially if she didn't have to worry about her mother anymore. All this is important for the therapist to keep in mind throughout the beginning stage, and to even be willing to say aloud in order to counter the possible fantasies, especially for Ms. Harris. The mother needs to hear that the therapist doesn't need to take over like Ellen is trying to do, but can support her in making the shifts she as the parent needs to make.

Ellen didn't come back in, but instead sat the rest of the session in the waiting room. The therapist spent the rest of the time giving Ms. Harris and the other two girls some feedback—empathizing with their sadness and the change in the family, pointing out their different coping styles, including Ellen's, and underscoring their secret feelings—the way Betsy worried about her mother, the way Marie missed her father, the way Ms. Harris worried about the children. The therapist also gave them permission to talk about their feelings, to talk about their father openly at home, to ask questions, to bring it all out in the open. Both girls agreed to come back at another time. At the end of the session the therapist then went out and talked to Ellen; she agreed to come in a talk to the therapist individually.

As with Billy we're at the fork in the path. Several options are open to us, depending upon your theoretical frame of reference, including staying with whole family therapy so that Betsy and Marie are not excluded. But if it's true that Ms. Harris needs to be the fulcrum of change, she may need some individual work to set her on course. Likewise, Ellen may have a easier time focusing upon her adolescent life if she doesn't have the rest of the family as an audience to ignite her role. The therapist decided to see if Ms. Harris could help facilitate grief work at home and to temporarily see her and Ellen separately.

ELLEN ALONE

When Ellen came in the following week, she looked anxious. The therapist suspected that she may have been a bit gun-shy from the family session, afraid that the therapist would once again start talking about her father.

Of course she didn't. Even alone she wouldn't have handled it any better and would only learn to dread therapy itself. Instead the therapist asked her about her school and social life, her friends and boyfriends and dreams about the future. Most of all the therapist wanted to listen while she talked not about her family, but her life as a teenager.

And she did. Perhaps it was the relief of not having to talk about something more difficult that spurred her on, or maybe she was feeling more comfortable with the therapist and dropping her tough exterior. It doesn't matter why, so much as that she was able to step out of her role, show her other side and inner life, and be supported and encouraged for doing so.

The session ended with the therapist thanking her for talking, and, much as he had at the end of the last session with her mother and sisters, empathizing with the changes she and the family had faced. The therapist worried aloud that Ellen had taken on too much responsibility, that everybody else in the family saw her as mean and angry, but that they didn't really know how she felt or what her world was like. Of course, Ellen had to agree with her because this is what she just spent the session talking about (explanation follows experience). The therapist suggested that she would like to help her be a better teenager and help her worry less about her mother and sisters.

Ellen said little, but seemed much more relaxed. Essentially, the therapist was giving her permission to step down. This didn't mean she automatically would or could—there was still a lot of power in her role, a need for her behavior to maintain the family patterns, and the underlying grief driving it all. But if Ms. Harris could begin to take up the slack, the new space within the family structure could be created for Ellen, and perhaps then she could be able to grieve. Ellen agreed to meet alone with the therapist a couple of more times, think about specific things she would like help with, and meet with mother again in a few weeks.

TALKING TYPES

In contrast to sessions with young children, these individual sessions with an adolescent are different simply because of the age difference. Whereas the play becomes the medium for Billy, the means for projecting and healing his inner world, talking becomes the medium for Ellen. Ellen's role and maturity made this easy for her.

But not all adolescents are as vocal as Ellen. In fact, adolescents are notorious for shutting down, sitting in the chair, grunting and staring at their shoes. Those, like Ellen, who are parentified, seem to be the most willing talkers. Because they sound so much like adults, the danger is in talking to them as though they are. Doing so not only reinforces their role and defenses, but lulls you into believing that they're more mature than they really are and encourages you to gloss over their developmental struggles. Rather than letting them talk on and on about their concerns about everyone else, you need to steer teenagers like this toward their underlying, less easily talked about feelings and concerns about being a teenager.

Some teens are able to do this easily and use the therapist as a confidant. You become the big sister or brother, the good, laid-back parent, their best friend's mother whom they like so much. April, for example, a 16-year-old, would easily and eagerly talk about how she felt left out of the cliques at school, self-conscious about her body, ambivalent toward her father. She wondered aloud about the purpose of religion, the materialism of our culture, heady but normal expressions of adolescent existentialism and angst. Her isolation made her hungry for the opportunity simply to communicate with someone whom she could trust, and through the process, in a Rogerian way, to discover who she is. Her trusting of the therapist became the template for trusting others around her.

Of course, some adolescents seem to be open like April, but the openness is really an anxiety-avoiding, rather than anxiety-facing, process. What they talk about is no different from what they talk with their best friends about on the phone every night. Sometimes this reflects their misunderstanding of just what therapy is about, how the conversation and the relationship is different from that with a peer. You have the responsibility to clarify your role and the purpose of the process—"Becky, I appreciate your telling me about your friends at school, but I'm not sure why you're telling me about it. What worries you the most? How can I help you with your feelings?" If it continues, then it is up to you to ask the deeper questions, and help the adolescent move toward what's missing in the process in order to create a new experience.

As with adults, there are important differences between adolescents who won't talk and those that can't talk, or at least can't talk well. James, a 14-year-old, was referred by his school principal because he was crudely propositioning girls in his class at school for sex. He and his mother came in together for the first session and were seen by a woman therapist. James said little in the session, and the therapist thought that James was reluctant to talk because it was the initial session, she was a woman, and his mother was present. So arrangements were made for James to be seen individually by a man on the staff.

Communication was still a struggle. James never initiated conversation and would only answer questions with the fewest words possible. When the therapist tried to talk to James about his sexuality ("So, James, what do you think about girls?"), the communication, although it didn't seem possible, broke down even more. The therapist then tried to talk about the apparent problem of talking ("James, it seems that talking about all these things seems really hard for you"), but this got nowhere. The therapist felt discouraged.

It was only after the therapist received records from the school that he discovered that James had an IQ of 80. James's difficulty communicating may have reflected some of his resistance or embarrassment, but, the therapist realized, it probably reflected a communication problem on his side as well. James couldn't fully understand what the therapist was asking because he was probably talking over the boy's head. The therapist needed to talk more concretely and ask more specific questions ("Did you think that girl liked you?") to help James articulate what he was thinking and feeling. This painstaking process itself was valuable because it was James's difficulty appropriately expressing himself that led to the presenting problem.

But there are some adolescents who sound like James who are refusing to talk. They may have been dragged in by the parents, ordered to come by the court, or referred by the school, and they want no part of it. Someone else has the problem, not them, and they see no reason to be there or to talk to another adult who is going to give them a hard time.

There are several ways of approaching a grunter like this. One of the best is to see him or her together with the whole or part of the family. This sidesteps the grueling one-on-one struggle. You can encourage one of the parents to talk with him, which is, after all, their job, not the therapist's. By your exploration of the entire family landscape the adolescent sees that the focus isn't only on him or her, and anxiety goes down. Better yet, usually someone in the family will say something outrageous enough to ignite some response from the teen. All you then have to do is give him or her the space to talk and be heard.

Another variation of the family session is to ask the teen to bring in a friend to the first family session. Sometimes these friends serve as advocates and help the teen speak up to the parents. But more often they confront the teen for keeping quiet or lying or doing self-destructive things like taking drugs or skipping school. Again, such confrontation has the effect of clearing the air quickly and getting the process moving.

Peer confrontation is, of course, the value of adolescent groups. The focus keeps moving around, and the comments of one are likely to spark responses in the others. If there are peers in the group who easily talk, and/or are familiar with the group process, they can be the cotherapists, and leave you out of the power struggle.

While most teens will generally warm up once they discover that you're different than their parents and teachers (better yet, that you have a sense of humor), are empathic to their point of view, and are interested in helping them change what they want to change, truly oppositional adolescents will cling to their corner of the ring at the slightest movement you make toward them. In that case some therapeutic aikido—"You know, if I were you I wouldn't say anything you don't want to say here, especially anything important"—is enough to challenge them to open up.

Some therapists prefer to move from the physical to the verbal. A quick game of Nerf basketball in the office or Frisbee outside, especially with boys or younger teens, at the beginning of the session burns up that initial anxiety, builds rapport (especially if you lose), and can break the tension. Playing cards while casually asking questions can provide something for the teen to focus on while thinking or getting anxious. Other clinicians (as did the psychiatrist portrayed by Robin Williams in the film *Good Will Hunting*) prefer to wait the adolescent out. After they map out the terrain of therapy, it's up to the adolescent to make the first move. The client's growing anxiety from the silence and the sitting usually is enough to start something. Other times it's fine to say that it's okay to be quiet here. Again, for the oppositional teen, it has a strategic effect and gets him or her to talk; for others it genuinely gives them a chance to settle in and collect their thoughts. What's important for the clinician is to avoid the power struggle, to convey the need not for compliance, but choice.

Finally, some adolescents who may clam up in front of parents or alone with the therapist (who seems like another parent) do well when paired with sibling. Invariably the quiet teen has a sibling who is not. This mini-family group not only gives the therapist a different perspective on family life, but the sibling at least provides something for both the therapist and adolescent to respond to—"Your sister and I were talking about

your Uncle Max last week. How do you get along with him?" This allows
the teen to wade into therapeutic waters on a buddy system. Once the adolescent feels more comfortable, generally within a session or at most two,
the sibling can be phased out and reappear again in whole family sessions.
What you do want to avoid is the teen becoming dependent upon his or
her brother or sister, allowing the sibling to be his or her voice, or reducing his or her anxiety by making the sibling the focus of therapy.[1]

Over the course of the two individual sessions Ellen was able to talk
about specific problems at home (Betsy's constant intrusion), as well as at
school (having an argument with her best friend). In each case the therapist helped her clarify what her feelings were (e.g., feeling rejected and
hurt by her friend) and *her* problem (e.g., Betsy's feeling bored is not Ellen's problem, but Betsy's). In each case she was encouraged not to be responsible for problems that are not hers (e.g., working harder than Betsy
to fix her boredom), and to be assertive toward her sisters, her mother,
and her friends, rather than suppressing her feelings or getting angry and
creating a cutoff.

While Ellen's problems were upsetting but overall relatively minor,
sometimes more serious problems are revealed in individual sessions. After a few sessions a teen may talk about heavy use of marijuana, reveal a
previously undisclosed incidence of sexual abuse, or admit to a two-year
history of bulimia, problems obviously overriding the initial treatment
plan. A more thorough substance abuse evaluation may be necessary; ethical and legal requirements mandate that protective services be notified of
the sexual abuse; further exploration is needed to map the triggers and
specific behaviors surrounding the eating disorder. Guidance from your
supervisor is essential. Impact on the therapeutic relationship, parent–
adolescent relationship, and therapeutic goals have to all be anticipated
and planned for. The focus shifts, new priorities are set, new contracts and
action plans need to be developed.

This was, fortunately, not the case with Ellen. The next week she was
able to report that she talked to her mother about Betsy, and had called up
her friend and worked things out.

---

[1]Ron Taffel has written a number of useful books for both clinicians and parents on dealing with
difficult teens in concrete ways in therapy and at home. See his *Breaking through to Teens*,
Guilford Press, 2005; *Getting through to Difficult Kids and Parents*, Guilford Press, 2000; *The Second
Family*, St. Martin's Griffin, 2002.

MS. HARRIS ALONE

Ellen's age, her ability, and her willingness to express herself and to think through realistic solutions to problems helped her take concrete steps at home and change the interactional patterns between her and her mother much more quickly and easily than Billy was able to do. When Ms. Harris was seen individually a couple of weeks later, she seemed less stressed; she reported that Ellen had been less demanding and angry, and actually had come and talked to her about Betsy.

Upon hearing such news it could be tempting for the therapist to let Ellen continue to take the lead and initiate the changes at home. But this would not only slow down the change process, but would re-create and maintain the reactive role that Ms. Harris had learned. In order for there to be long-term change in Ms. Harris and in her relationship with her other daughters, she needed to make individual changes herself.

The therapist asked her about her relationship with her husband. Once again she sighed and seemed to collapse, but then slowly was able to talk about her loss and the first edges of her anger. His alcoholism and his violent temper had overwhelmed her at times, and she admitted to retreating into a passive accommodation to avoid conflict. Relinquishing any intimate relationship with her husband, she made the children the focus of her concern and needs. When asked, she acknowledged feeling responsible in some way for his drinking and even his death. Perhaps she could have tried harder, helped him to get sober, made sure he had gone to the doctor for a checkup. If she had, she and the children wouldn't be where they are.

Even though she may not have voiced her guilt aloud before, the feelings themselves were familiar and part of the constellation of emotions that kept her in her passive, reactive role. Rather than letting her sink into these emotions yet again, the therapist stepped in and did some light education about alcoholism and grief, stating that feeling guilty and responsible are a normal part of both for families. There was silence for several minutes, then Ms. Harris shifted gears and talked about Ellen.

Ms. Harris had never used threats in an effort to make Ellen behaviorally comply, but many parents do. Those who view their teenager as the problem, and/or whose own frustrations have reached their limit, come to rely on threats as the only means they feel they have of controlling their child. Over and over the message to the adolescent, and to the therapist, is that the teen better shape up or else, the else usually being shipping the child out to foster care somewhere. Usually the threats don't work—the adolescent feels the power move and fights back, or feels the rejection and says he or she doesn't care.

Once you help the parents find other ways of responding to the adolescent's behavior the threat usually stops. But some parents need backing, need to know that the community, and not just the therapist, is behind them. This support can usually come through the schools, if the teen is having trouble there, or through the courts, if the adolescent is acting out in the community. The teachers, principal, or probation officer can be invited to come to meetings with the parent. They can clarify their role, their concern, their limits, and work with the parent to create a united front to the teen. The principal can stress the consequences of cutting school or offer rewards for completing work, the probation officer can let the teen know that he or she will personally bring the teen before the judge if he or she continues to ignore the parents' curfew. In many cases this is essential to keep the adolescent from splitting the adults and undermining the changes the parent is trying to make.

But even with this backing some parents still lapse into threats. Even when changes are occurring they let the teen and the therapist know that placement outside the home is always in their mind. This kind of talk can undermine the teen's willingness to work on changes, pull the process back into power struggles, and sabotage any sense of security.

One of the best ways I've found for handling the periodic making of such threats is to simply call the parent on it, that is, to take the parent's threat as a serious option. Whether you see this as a paradoxical move, a way of calling the parent's bluff, or a sincere acknowledgment of what the parent is saying, the outcome is the same. Saying something to the effect of "Mr. Neal, I've been hearing you say to Tom on and off for months now that if he doesn't change, you don't want to deal with him anymore. Maybe I haven't been taking your feelings seriously enough, and we need to talk about whether we should make plans for Tom to stay somewhere else for awhile."

The message here is that what you say will be believed, rather than minimized, that it's all right to consider placement if the parents need a break. By your taking a clear, strong stance, you not only draw out the issue of commitment and what it means to love someone, but provide a strong antidote to ambivalence. The clients are essentially pushed off the fence they have been sitting upon. Your clarity forces them to clarify their own position, and challenges them to match words with intent and to take responsibility for their feelings and decisions. The discussion can quickly tap into the parents' own history—the way their parents managed their adolescence.

The net effect of this type of confrontation is get all their feelings and intention clearly on the table, and help the parents separate threat and need for control from their true feelings. Most parents will recommit themselves to the process and stop the threats. But some may actually need to sort out their emotions and the possibility of the teen's planned leaving of the home. The therapist's job is to help the parent place this decision in a context and to make it a decision, rather than a frustrated reaction.

Ms. Harris had already demonstrated in her marriage a high tolerance for turmoil and so, not surprisingly, had never reached this point with Ellen. The therapist used the sessions with the mother to map out, with role playing and brainstorming, specific responses for specific situations that she could use should Ellen become too demanding or out of control. To offset the mother's greater setting of limits, they also talked about ways she could spend more quality time with Ellen and new, different ways Ellen could help her at home, creating for Ellen (and herself) a new role to replace what was being taken away.

By focusing on Ms. Harris's parenting skills, on what she as the mother could do, rather than her tales of victimization or on what was wrong with Ellen, the session experience was one of empowerment, the goal one of action rather than reaction and helplessness. By not moving too quickly and overloading her, by staying alert to her becoming too passive and merely accommodating the therapist, Ms. Harris could be led to have success experiences at home that could help her see herself as a capable parent.

RETURN OF THE FAMILY

After three individual sessions each with Ms. Harris and Ellen, home life was beginning to calm down. Although she could easily fall back to her old ways when she was under stress, Ms. Harris was more and more able to set limits with Ellen. She found, to her amazement, that Ellen, after a lot of initial huffing and puffing, was willing to do as she asked. And Ellen spoke of spending time with her mother alone, something that she had not done in years, and hadn't realized how much she had missed.

It was time to bring the rest of the family back in, to find out the impact of these changes on the other girls, and to see what effect it was all having on the family's grief reaction. So in they trooped again, this time Betsy leading the line straggling down the hall, with Ellen and Ms. Harris walking together, taking up the rear. Ms. Harris sat by herself in a chair with Ellen on one couch next to her and Betsy and Marie together on the other. Betsy seemed a bit less rambunctious than last time, and her mother asked her to take her feet off the cushion. Marie still seemed quiet and depressed.

After touching base with Betsy and Marie ("How have you been?" "How was the field trip you told me about last time?"), the therapist asked about how things have been going at home. True to form Betsy immediately piped up that Ellen had not been fighting so much.

"And you like that?" asked the therapist.

Betsy nodded her head. Ms. Harris smiled. "And Ellen even let me borrow her sweatshirt."

"You looked like a dork," said Ellen with a smile. "It went all the way down to your knees."

"It wasn't quite her size," chimed in Ms. Harris, "but it was nice of Ellen to let her use it." Ms. Harris looked at Ellen and smiled; Ellen smiled back.

The hierarchy had shifted. Ellen and Betsy were relating more as siblings. Ms. Harris was more in charge and positive toward Ellen. Marie, however, was still quiet.

"How about for you, Marie? Things feel any different at home? Not having to hide out in your room so much?"

"Yeah, I guess," she said flatly.

"How are you and Ellen getting along?"

"Okay."

"I asked her to come to the mall with me the other night, but she didn't want to go," said Ellen.

"Marie and I talked some the other night," said Ms. Harris. "I think she is still having a hard time about her dad."

Marie's eyes began to water.

"Is what your mom is saying true? Have you been missing your dad a lot?"

Marie nodded her head.

"I bet it has still been hard for all of you." The therapist looked around the room, making eye contact with everyone.

"We went to his grave this past Sunday and brought flowers" said Betsy. "I felt sad."

"We hadn't gone in a long time. I decided we needed to do that," said Ms. Harris.

The mother again was taking charge. Ellen so far was staying in her chair, didn't seem to be getting anxious or angry. The goal now was to help everyone in the family stay with the process and help allow the emotions to come out. The content itself wasn't important; it was only a medium for the emotions.

"Marie, how did you feel at the cemetery?"

"Sad." She was on the verge of tears.

"I picked the flowers," said Betsy.

Betsy was trying to distract from the emotions to help Marie. Appropriately, the mother reached over and gently touched Betsy's knee and put her finger to her lips. Betsy leaned back and got quiet. Ellen was staring at Marie.

"What do you miss most about your dad, Marie?" asked the therapist, quietly.

"I miss going with him on Sunday mornings to get the paper." Her voice was barely audible, and tears were welling up.

"If your Dad were sitting here right now," said the therapist as she pulled an empty chair alongside of her, "what would you say to him?"

"I'd say that . . . " Marie started quietly crying. Ms. Harris was tearing up, as was Ellen. Betsy was sitting quietly with her head down.

"I—" started Betsy, but Ms. Harris reached over and touched her knee again. Betsy leaned back again and was quiet.

The only sounds in the room were the sniffling and crying of everyone. The therapist said quietly that it seemed that everyone had been feeling sad for a while and missing their father, and that it had been hard to talk about, and probably was making everyone feel lonely. Again the goal was to facilitate the process, not to interpret. In contrast to the last family session, everyone was able to stay in the room together.

After several minutes Ms. Harris spoke: "I think it would be good for us if we took out the old family videos sometime this week and looked at them." Everyone nodded.

"I remember when we all went out West," said Betsy.

"Do you remember that? Harris said. "You were so young."

"I remember Dad went horseback riding with us and almost fell off," Ellen said, half smiling.

"Yeah, he had that huge horse. My head was up to its knee," Marie said.

"I think we have movies of that," said Harris. "We'll have to get them out."

Everyone talked about things that they most remember, including Ellen's bringing up of Dad's temper. The therapist guided the process and helped clarify the emotions, asking about other memories and emotions: "What was the happiest time?" "Who felt scared when Dad got mad?" "Can you picture him now?" "It hurts, doesn't it?" Drawing out these details brought the emotions to the surface, and kept everyone from veering off defensively.

The therapist also asked if anyone felt that it was their fault that their dad got so angry or even that he died. There was a long, awkward silence which Ms. Harris then filled by saying to the children that it wasn't their fault, that their father drank too much, and that this made his anger worse. His drinking, and his death, she said, to them, to herself, had nothing to do with them.

Each member of the family was sorting through her grief. Like Billy finally remembering and talking about his brother's death, this session too was the opening up of the process, not the end of it. This family would need to have more talks like this, more open sharing of feelings as they together and individually worked through the loss. But now that Ms. Harris was empowered, she could serve as a role model for the children of the grief process. Now that they could feel that she could support them, and they, in turn, no longer needed to feel responsible for taking care of her, the natural healing process could follow its course.

WRAPPING UP

The family met again the following week, and again it was a mixture of emotion and recollection. The family talked about seeing the family videos, everyone related once again some past memories, but they were also able to shift focus and talk about solving day-to-day problems—Who was going to cook when Ms. Harris had to work late one night?—with the mother taking charge. At the end of session, it was decided that Ms. Harris and Ellen would each come in individually one more time.

The session with Ellen felt like one of those termination sessions where there seemed to be not much to talk about, no strong pressure to resolve anything. Ellen mostly talked about school, her plans to get a job over the summer, her hope to visit Disney World with one of her friends and her family. The session ended with an agreement that she could come back by herself anytime she wanted.

The session with Ms. Harris was a debriefing of the family sessions, a review of all the positive changes she had been making, with the therapist clearly in the role of consultant. All the changes in patterns were reviewed, and ways of keeping the door open on the grief process and supporting Marie were discussed. What was most striking about Ms. Harris was her strength, her assertiveness. Like Ellen, she too was told to feel free to come back anytime by herself, with the entire family, or with one of the kids.

Of course, there are other avenues that this therapist and family could have followed—more individual work with Ms. Harris, ongoing monitoring of Ellen, sessions with Ellen and Ms. Harris, individual work with Marie to help her with her sadness, continued family sessions to help them possibly unravel more of their anger and solidify the changes in the family structure. All these options, no doubt, have merit and might have helped this family.

But therapy can and often should end with significant but modest changes. This family had moved beyond that place they were stuck. They are on a solid, more developmentally appropriate path. They learned some skills (particularly the mom) that they should be able to use as they individually and together face the changes and challenges to come in the next few years. If, after these sessions, they were still lumbering under their grief—if the mother was unable to develop more power in spite of the therapist's coaching, if Ellen remained angry or shifted her anger to another arena (for example, started fighting at school or ran away), if Marie or Betsy stepped in to take Ellen's place as the I.P. and began to have severe symptoms that Ms. Harris could not help them with, more work would obviously be needed.

Some families are content merely getting to the other side of a crisis; others want therapy to leave them with a firmer sense of stability and some new skills; while still others, building on the momentum of the initial changes, want to continue in order to maximize the family's potential. Where the end is located is determined by your and their expectations for therapy. What you don't want is to leave them feeling fragile, of desiring and needing more help and not getting it, of resolving the initial problem, but being left staring at the one or several that have taken its place.

Why did this case turn out seemingly better than that with Billy? Probably because the trauma was not so great, because Ellen at her age was able to verbalize her feelings and direct her behavior more deliberately perhaps, because Ms. Harris's level of depression wasn't as great as Billy's grandmother's and she didn't feel as isolated. In addition, the therapists were different, in their personality, their clinical strengths and weaknesses, their ability to join with the family—101 variables that affect the course and outcome of a case that are beyond anyone's awareness or direct control. This, of course, is part of what makes for the art of therapy and the challenges that come with each new case.

Looking Within: Chapter 12 Exercises

Adolescence is a bridge between two different worlds. During those few short years we consolidate and build on the lessons learned in childhood about ourselves and life. We are forced to look ahead to our future and our "grown-up" selves while struggling to discover who we are in the present. How well we master the challenges of adolescence and learn the lessons that it needs to teach us often becomes the template upon which we shape our adulthood for years to come. As you do these exercises, think back and remember your life as a teenager.

1. Think about your own attitudes about adolescents. Should they, in general, be given more freedom, more discipline? What does your answer tell you about what you believe adolescents need to learn most?

2. How might a therapist have been helpful to you when you were a teenager? How would have individual therapy been useful?

Family therapy? What would have been your attitude toward each? How would have your family reacted?

3. In what situations, with what types of problems or families with teenagers are you apt to overidentify, project, resist?

4. How might have a psychoanalyst, a Rogerian individual therapist, a biologically oriented psychiatrist have handled the case of the Harris family differently? What do you see as the major advantages or disadvantages of each?

5. Comparing the contrasting cases involving younger children and teens, which do you feel more confident about? What specific skills do you most need to develop?

6. How do you privately decide just how good a job you are doing with a particular family?

[13]

Getting to the Core
COUPLE WORK IN FAMILY THERAPY

The room seems empty, and quiet. It's just you, Eric, and Cathy. No kids, no fighting over blocks, Play-Doh, or puppets; no stretching out of a parent's arm to rein in one child before he has a chance to go clobber his brother. You're wondering what they did with the kids (stuffed them in the trunk of the car? Dropped them off at Grandma's?) to come alone, but then you decide you really don't want to know.

Your mission: To help this couple gain some control over the bedlam at home. With four children between the ages of four and 12, two of them at any one time are fighting in some sort of a tag-team arrangement. Actually, this should be pretty simple: Find out where things break down, help the parents clarify their rules and their responses, make sure they are working together as a team. Straightforward child management.

"So how was your week?" you casually throw out to give yourself time to grab your coffee cup behind you and settle in.

"Didn't I send him to his room, didn't I?" Cathy snaps. "I specifically told Danny to stay in his room for 10 minutes."

Whoa, did you just miss something, you wonder, as you barely swallow your first sip of coffee.

Eric, nervously pulling on his shirt collar, apparently knows what Cathy is talking about. "Then three minutes later he's out there in kitchen with me, telling me that *you* told him his time-out was over!" Frail, quiet Cathy of last week suddenly is sounding angry and tough. She's now glaring at Eric, who is taking a deep breath and getting ready to swing into his defense.

" I thought you were being too hard on him, I—"

"But you do this all the time, Eric, ALL THE TIME!" Now she's getting hot.

"No, I *don't* do this all the time." Eric's cranking up too. "You're the one who always lets Allison off easy, but do I say anything about it? No, I don't, because—

"Don't give me that. I don't treat her any different than the boys. I'm the one—"

So much for a quiet, peaceful session.

Most families enter therapy around problems with children, and, as we've discussed in previous chapters, your assessment involves understanding the dysfunctional family patterns, the skill base of the parents, the individual needs of the children, the environmental stressors. As with Billy's grandmother, Ms. Harris, and now Cathy and Eric, some portion of your work may involve working alone with the parent or parents to build skills and shift roles. This approach, however, is different from the one that therapists who are not trained to work with children are often tempted to make, namely, to assume that all the real issues in families lie within the couple relationship of two adults.

Essentially, such clinicians, it seems, have learned that they can relieve their anxiety about what to do with the kids by taking a reductionistic approach: See the family for a couple of sessions, uncover some marital problem, throw the kids out, and focus instead on this smaller, more manageable unit. Yes, the couple may do better (or not), the children may do better (or not). But as has been said before, family therapy is not about the number of people in the room, but a way of thinking about the source and solution to problems. If you find that your goals are only about improving the couple's adult relationship and you are no longer thinking about the family, kids, parenting, you're probably no longer doing family therapy.

All that being said, it is valuable to think about the dynamics of the couple in the context of the family therapy. Just as it is helpful to create for yourself and the family a vision of how they together would want to be, it's helpful to create your own vision of how the couple ideally needs to be. Good communication, respect, flexibility. Good problem-solving and decision-making skills. A united front with the kids, a willingness to compromise, a commitment to each other and their parental relationship.

An ability to separate out their issues as a couple from those of the children, to see themselves as the building block, the central core of the family—all these readily come to mind. Basically, when the couple is sound, the rest of the family is sound.

But when the couple is not, things begin to fall apart. When the rules become unclear or contradictory, the children wind up either constantly testing as a way of defining them, or ignoring them. When the parents aren't united, the children quickly learn to split them—bypass the tough one and ask the easy one, or appeal to the other if you don't like what the first one said. When problems are never solved or communication is poor, the household is in a state of tension as the same problems come up over and over again. When the parents are always battling or struggling with each other the tension is magnified, and the kids learn to lean on each other for support, withdraw or escape, or (especially young children) blame themselves for what they believe is happening.

DANGEROUS STRUCTURES

When such patterns become part of the fabric of the couple relationship, when the battles are not just simple differences of opinion, but relentless struggles for power, or worse, when tensions are never openly expressed, but instead are driven underground, the entire family structure becomes warped and distorted. This distortion can take various overlapping forms, varying in their toxicity and effect on the children:

The Child-Centered Family

Many parents, usually following core values of their culture, often make their children their primary focus and essentially believe that children come first. Such families can be healthy and happy because the parents can have a good relationship with each other even if they spend more of their energy on the children than we as therapists or as the mass American culture feel comfortable with. This is very different from the child-centered families often seen in therapy offices. In these families there is a breakdown of the couple relationship, a longing for a different type of relationship or a return to an earlier and better time, an awareness that the children have become the glue and focus holding them together. You can ask questions like "Which one of you is more likely to want to spend a little less time on the children and a little more time on each other?" and see where the question leads.

Generally this breakdown happens over a period of years. Imagine the start of marriage being like moving into a new, large house. There's room to explore, places to decorate and make your own, space to move around. But over the years the rooms become dusty and dirty and slowly filled with junk—resentments, half-finished arguments, unexpressed needs, memories of hurt. Rather than getting up the courage and cleaning these rooms out by talking about what is difficult to say, one by one the couple simply shuts and locks the rooms. Over and over this happens through the years until the once beautiful and large house seems narrow and cramped as the couple finds themselves living in the hallway by the front door. The only safe topics are the weather and that no-good supervisor on the job; the only safe focus at home is the kids. Even though both may occasionally look at each other and shift their eyes upstairs, they just as quickly glance away. The couple silently makes a pact to be good parents, if not good lovers.

There are two dangers that arise from this structure. One is that the children of such parents will by default use this as a model of their own couple relationships and families. Even though they have a strong model for parenting, they lack one for adult intimacy. As coupled adults they may think they are doing the right things, but wonder why they feel empty or awkward when they are alone without children. Essentially how they wind up feeling is just the same as their parents did, but which the latter, as children, were never aware of. They have failed to learn that being an adult in all its roles and forms is something valuable in its own right.

The other danger is that anxiety, even panic, can set in as the children begin to leave home and the parents face the prospect of being alone with just themselves. They may either undermine the children's leaving ("Why don't you go to the college right here in town, Dear?") or scramble to find other replacements (for example, adopting children, acquiring pets; becoming workaholic or alcoholic, and so on) to fill in the holes. It's usually a good idea to ask parents of teens at some point what they are most looking forward to once the kids leave home. If they say not much because they expect that the kids will be living right around the corner, or Dad says he's planning on spending most of the winter in his fishing shack up on the lake, you have a good sense of possible couple-transition distress.

Separate Lives

At the next level of distortion the split between the couple becomes wider and the parenting pact collapses. Rather than being solved with children, the problem of intimacy is solved with distance. In such families one of the parents is often *the* parent (commonly the mother), while the other is somewhere else (at work, outside in the garage, out with friends). In other families the parents take turns—one minds the kids certain days or parts of days while the other is off, and then they switch. There isn't so much conflict as emptiness, deadness. The children are involved with one parent, the other is gone, and rarely do the children have a chance to see how the parents interact with each other. In their own couple relationships as adults the children re-create these patterns and struggle with the same emotions.

The Surrogate Partner

Of course, a parent's intimacy needs can also be met through one of the children. It's normal and healthy for parents and children to have close relationships, but this closeness becomes unhealthy when the hierarchal boundaries become blurred. In its most extreme form we find physical incest, where a parent literally co-opts one of the children to be his or her mate. But there can also be varying degrees of emotional incest as well, such as when a parent starts complaining to his or her child about the other parent, or uses the child as a confidant of money troubles or the current romantic relationship. The child is treated more as a adult than a child, and plays out an adult role in the parent's life.

When this type of blurring occurs we often wind up with a child or teenager with a sense of entitlement and distorted sense of power, an overresponsibility for a parent or the family, and a loss at some level of his or her own childhood. Rather than struggling to retain a place in the relationship, the other parent may physically leave, emotionally leave by essentially taking on a role as one of the kids, or form a coalition with the rest of the kids against the other parent and the favorite child.[1]

---

[1] In many of these structures it is interesting to see how they are unconsciously displayed in the simple sitting arrangement of the family in the session—the kids literally filling the space on the couch between the two parents, the surrogate sitting next to the "partner" parent, with the other parent across the room in the corner. Asking family members to change seats can raise anxiety but help change the dynamics in the room.

Ganging Up

Coalitions and collusions with children by one parent against the other aren't so much driven by a lack of marital intimacy as much as by anger. Rather than acknowledging each parent's separate sphere of power (e.g., work vs. parenting), or, as in the child-centered family, accepting at some level the lack of a relationship, here the children are always triangled into an unending marital struggle. The mother becomes the ringleader of the children against mean old Dad; Dad heads up the gang of boys in the family against Mom and Sally. Arguments may be over parenting, but it is all projection ("Stop picking on Tommy; let him do what he wants!" rather than saying "Let me do what I want"). The conflict may be open or subtle, but, regardless, the effect is one of splitting the family into camps, with each side against the other. Once you are aware of the process, get the parent ringleaders to talking and speaking for themselves.

Sibling Rivalry: Fighting by Proxy

Some sibling rivalry in families is be expected. Not only do children get irritable with each other just as adults do, but every child also wants to feel special in the eyes of the parents, and so at times inevitably feels jealous or resentful of the other sibling. Generally, children can learn to work these conflicts out on their own. If the parents interfere too much in their squabbles they can inadvertently reinforce them—the children learn that one way to get the parents' attention is to start a fight.

In families where the parents openly argue, the children may take ordinary sibling rivalry one step further. Copying the parents' models of interaction the children argue and fight most of the time. The parents may do little to stop it because they are so caught up in the marital conflict, or may foster the children's fighting by taking sides.

When the parents fight by proxy, the children do the fighting for the parents and express the anger and conflict that the parents cannot. There may be tension between the parents but rarely open conflicts; they may acknowledge differences between them, but seem unable or unwilling to settle them. They often come to you concerned about the constant bickering among the children. The parents seem helpless to stop it; attempts are half-hearted or are undermined by the parents' inability to work together as a unit. Their own frightening anger, lying just below the surface, keeps them from getting clear and organized enough to be effective.

The problem and the patterns, like most negative patterns with children, continue because essentially everyone wins: The children have emotional outlets and means of gaining, if not positive attention, at least negative attention from the parents; the parents have vicarious outlets for their own anger, as well as a comfortable, familiar problem around which to focus their anxiety.

As with other parenting issues, those of sibling rivalry need to be tracked in terms of knowledge and skill and patterns. I usually begin by asking parents what their expectations are. If a parent, for example, has trouble tolerating any conflict at all, the question is why: Was he or she an only child, perhaps, and has no experience with normal sibling interactions? Was sibling conflict not tolerated in his or her childhood home, through repressive measures? Does any conflict somehow reflect negatively on the parental self-image? Does the parent become anxious and uncertain how to respond concretely?

If the tolerance seems extremely high (siblings are physically hurt or emotionally abused), is it an acting out of the couple's anger or the couple's relationship, a parent's seeming unawareness due to depression or other emotional preoccupation, or a parent's an inability to act due to a lack of skill?

Rather than stepping in too late, too heavy-handed, or not at all, I suggest to parents that they try and take a preventive approach. Give the kids positive feedback when they are interacting well ("You guys are playing so well together with your trucks!"). Keep an ear out for the beginnings of conflict, and if it sounds like it is beginning to escalate, try distracting or separating ("Tony, would you come and help me make dinner?"). Be clear about rules (e.g., you can get mad but no hitting) and consequences, and talk about the process after everyone is calm ("How come you guys were fussing with each other before? How can you both fix the problem?").[2] If the parents can't follow through with these suggestions, you need to look at breaking down the suggestions into smaller, more manageable and understandable pieces, or wonder about their need for problem as a solution.

---

[2]The classic book for parents on managing sibling rivalry is Adele Faber, *Siblings Without Rivalry*, Collins, 2004.

All of these patterns—the ganging up, the children as surrogates, the child centered relationship, the fighting by proxy—distort the parent–child relationship by placing children in inappropriate roles that threaten their security and trample their development. The patterns are easily formed because of the children's malleability and dependency on the parents. In exchange for some attention and sense of purpose they take on habits and roles that re-create the parents' own pasts or fill holes in the sinking marital relationship. Like other patterns, they interlock and quickly become entrenched. Even if one of the parents attempts to change the process of the family relationships, he or she may run not only into a power struggle with the other parent, but into resistance by the children, who become anxious by the change.

SEPARATING ROLES: ASSESSING THE COUPLE

This resistance doesn't mean that one parent (or even one child) can't bring about change in the family; they can, because a shift in one pattern will, with enough time and persistence, ripple through the others. But when the parents can separate their problems as a couple from those problems as parents, agree on what those problems are, and work together to present a united front to the children, changes can occur more quickly and can be sustained more easily.

In order to help the parents learn how to distinguish their needs and concerns as a couple from those as parents, you need to shift through and separate the roles and emotional dynamics that make up their relationship. Here's a quick checklist of questions to ask yourself and/or them:

• *Are couple problems defined?* Occasionally you will run across couples who state up front that it's their relationship that's creating problems in the family—they can't ever agree about the kids and their marital problems are making the kids upset. Such openness allows you to zero in on these issues and clearly improves the prognosis. When the child is the I.P., however, such couple problems may only be hinted at through side comments or joking remarks—"I think Carlos would settle down if she would just support me sometimes"; "Of course, I don't get any help with this—he's never home!" Picking up on these comments—"So you feel you need more support from your wife?" or "If your husband was around more, do you think it would help Carlos do better?"—is enough to open the door and get the couple talking about their relationship.

Oftentimes, however, they will polarize over the significance of their relationship and its impact on the children—one feels that the state of their relationship is the heart and soul of the family problems, while the other believes it has absolutely nothing to do with the kids. The problems are being replicated right there in the room, and you can sometimes start with that: "It seems like you have a difference of opinion about whether this is important enough to bring up. Sam, maybe you can tell Maria why you think it is?" or "Maria, Sam's bringing up things that you'd rather not talk about and that seems to bother you. Does this happen a lot?"

However you choose to ask the question, your interest is not about content but about process—you want to open the communication between the couple. You want to help them to define the terrain of their relationship, and by doing so in your presence and with your supportive response, learn that it is safe to do so. Once this is done, using the principle of explanation follows experience, you can then link this interaction to their concern about the presenting problem—"It sounds to me, from what you both have just said, that you both feel that the other one totally disregards what you say. I wonder if Carlos can sense this and uses the split between you to try and get his own way?" The link between the couple issues and parenting issues now seem more clear, and the couple is more motivated to explore their problems.

• *What emotions are presented and how are they handled?* Sarah is seething throughout the session while her husband Mike scarcely responds and seems depressed. Or perhaps both parents are flat and detached and the children do all the talking.

It's safe to assume that the process you see in your office replicates to some degree what happens at home. You want to notice not only the mood of each partner, but the mood in relationship to the other and perhaps the children. Does Mike always seem depressed and unresponsive, or is it his way of coping with Sarah's anger? Does he cope through alcohol or drugs? Does one of the children act out his anger? Does Sarah get angry because Mike is depressed? Is this her way of trying to get him to respond, or is it some internal response independent of Mike or anyone else? How else does she manage her emotions—through drugs, eating, having affairs?

Are the parents detached most of time, leaving the children to essentially take care of themselves? Are the children endlessly trying to find better ways of getting their parents to respond to them? How does any of this possibly tie into the presenting problem? For example, does Mike's depression make it easy for Michelle to walk all over Sarah? Does Jeff boss the other kids around because he feels like the parents aren't going to parent?

Through this brainstorming you are attempting to link the emotional lives of both the individual parents and of the couple as a unit with the rest of the family and the presenting problems. You can check out your hunches by directly asking questions to the couple: "Sarah, you seem angry. How do you feel about the fact that Mike is saying nothing back?" or "Mike, you seem depressed. Do you feel sometimes feel this way at home? Sarah, is this how Mike seems to feel around you at home?"

Again, your immediate goal is to open the communication. You want to explore both the emotional outlets and each partner's emotional flexibility. You want to track the way emotions bounce off each other and drive the behavioral patterns (e.g., Mike feels depressed and withdraws, Sarah feels overwhelmed by the children and gets angry, causing the children to run to Mike and drag him back into the family's interactions), and fuel the presenting problem (e.g. Jeff acts out Mike's anger toward Sarah). You're looking for where emotions need to be expanded (e.g., Mike needs to get in touch with his anger), where emotional triggers can be used by the couple as signals of a dysfunctional pattern (e.g., when Sarah starts to get angry Mike needs to step in rather than ignore her), and how to help the couple once again see how their moods spill out over each other and the rest of the family.

• *How has the relationship changed?* Explore changes in interaction (less affection, more affection, more arguments), changes in individual moods or personality (she's more irritable, he's more controlling), changes over time (how are they different from when they first met), and changes in the family (environmental, situational stress).

You are tracking two issues through these questions. The first is understanding how the needs of each partner for the other have changed over time. The developmental view of relationships tells us that all relationships naturally change over time because the people naturally continue to grow. Problems arise because there is a lag between these individual changes and the established rules, routines, and roles of the relationship. The woman, for example, who married someone who was a take-charge type of guy like her dad may resent the control 10 years later because that initial need was fulfilled over the time. Similarly, the man who married a woman who desperately needed him now feels weighed down with responsibilities and begins to resent her dependency. But the roles and routines created over the years are powerful, and only increase the frustration.

Rather than directly working to bring the relationship contract up to date, the couple may struggle over problems with children, or one or both of the individuals may act out (e.g., have an affair, go on shopping or drinking binges). The challenge is to reshape the relationship so that it can better represent the individuals within it.

But relationships not only changed from inside, but from outside sources as well. Even the strongest relationships have deteriorated or collapsed by the impact of serious illnesses, death of a child or other family member, job change or financial stress, even the building of a new house. Although it's tempting to see these stressors as only pushing on cracks already established in the foundation of the relationship, it's also reasonable to believe that a reduction of stress can get the relationship back on course.

• *How are decisions made about children, money, household chores, sex, and family outings and entertainment?* Most couples have, without openly discussing or even being aware of them, evolved rules and roles for making decisions between them. To ask couples how they make decisions is to make them and you aware of how the decision-making process itself works. You are also exploring power in the relationship—who is charge of what, who has the last word. Questions about parenting, money, sex, and household chores are the most common power issues in the family. Rather than finding a fair or effective solution to a problem ("Why don't you pay the rent from your check and I'll pay the child care from mine") gives way to battles over who's way is going to come out on top ("It's my money and you aren't going to tell me what to do with it").

Needless to say, these decision-making questions can arouse anxiety in the session and in the couple, and so it's important to consider your pacing. Hold off if the couple is wary or hostile of therapy itself, is clearly untrusting or still uncomfortable with you, or is already so anxious that anymore stress is likely to make them head for the door or shut up. But you shouldn't be reactive and wait for them to raise the issue.

Once they seem committed and settled, ask matter-of-factly how decisions are made and how disagreements are ended (someone gives in;

someone walks away and it's not discussed anymore; someone becomes violent). You want to help them become curious about the limits of their anger and ability to compromise, the underlying power structure and struggle, and the emotions that fuel them. Resentments that have been tucked away within these issues and which warp the family structure are often exposed. More importantly, perhaps, by raising these issues and their anxiety you're testing the waters. You're able to see right there and then how this couple will respond to the anxiety of change itself, where they may resist, how quickly or carefully you may have to go.

• *What is the role of children in the patterns of the couple?* How child-centered is the couple? Are children pulled into arguments literally or figuratively? Are the children divided in their support of the parents? Is one child a surrogate partner? Which parent spends what time with which child? How is the hierarchy skewed?

Again, by asking yourself these questions you are mapping the ways the children may become part of the couple's conflicts and solutions. By asking the partners some of these questions—What do the kids do when you argue? Do any of the kids join in and take sides? Which of the children do you think feels closest to your husband, to you?—you are once again beginning to link the couple's dynamics to the children's behaviors, helping them see where the children may be inappropriately being brought into their relationship.

• *How has the couple stabilized around the presenting problem?* In the 1980s there was a controversy in the family therapy field over whether people manufacture problems out of some neurotic need for stability; ultimately the field came to reject the notion. Most people's problems are oppressive, and people would do anything to rid of them. Nevertheless, problems arise, and families and couples often stabilize themselves around the existence of certain problems. This stability can serve as an impediment to addressing the problems directly.

Denise's drug use, for example, creates enough of an ongoing crisis and distraction that the couple argues about how to handle her rather than arguing about the ways they treat each other in the marriage. The answer to this question about the role of the problem in the family tells you what you may need to work on in the relationship if the presenting problem were to solidly change (e.g., the couple would need to acknowledge their conflicts; they would need to find positive rather than negative ways of interacting). Usually you can find clues to the answer right within the session process, such as when Denise acts up and distracts just at the point that tension arises between the couple, or the way the father switches topics to complain about Denise when you ask him a sensitive question about the marital relationship.

• *How severe are the relationship problems?* Have there been separations, divorce action, abuse, arrests, affairs? What's the worse their arguments have ever gotten? What you are trying to learn through these questions are the chronicity of the problems and patterns, the prognosis for the relationship, the need to focus on these issues before expecting any lasting change in other family patterns. Some couples will be upfront about this information, but many won't. If they seem reluctant, help them understand why you are asking, connect it the presenting problem, and show sensitivity, gentleness, and a sense of concern rather than judgment.

All these questions are similar to those you used in assessing the entire family, and, as you did with the family, you are looking to uncover both the couple's relationship structure and process. You are trying to learn whether problems have a way of being solved; whether change, even though difficult, can be accommodated; whether emotions have appropriate outlets; whether the couple is able to see their relationship as different from that of the children; and whether they both have a commitment to it and each other. By asking yourself these questions you can begin to separate out the couple from the family and can see by their response just how open they are to such exploration. By asking the couple these questions you are letting them know that their relationship is important in itself, is linked to the presenting problem, and vital to its solution.

CHOOSE YOUR FORMAT

How you gather and use what you learn will once again depend upon your own theoretical frame, your therapeutic style, and the expectations of the family. For example, some clinicians routinely use genograms as a way to both map the couple's history and family patterns (e.g., divorce is rampant as a solution to marital problems; grandmothers and granddaughters are close, but mothers and daughters are not) and help the couple see how larger patterns take hold within their relationship. Many clinicians matter-of-factly start in this manner: "I've found that sometimes parents have trouble making decisions (or handling a particular child, or getting along, etc.) because they have learned through their families different ways of approaching problems and relationships. I'd like to take a few minutes in this session to better understand some of your family background and what you've learned about parenting and solving problems. I'm going to ask you a few questions about your grandparents and parents and draw a map of it, which we can then look at together and compare."

The process of doing the genogram, as well as the product itself, allows the couple to step back and adapt a larger, more objective view of their problems. Rather than each feeling that the partner is out to get him or her, they become curious about the way they are both helping history to repeat itself.

On the other hand, a communications perspective looks not to history but to the skills the individuals need in order to express without attacking what they want their partner to know. The therapist will teach the couple how to make "I" statements, to discuss feelings rather than use rationalizations, to say what they want rather than what they don't like. This works well not only when communication is clearly poor, but when the less-threatening idea of "learning communication skills" can make the couple less anxious and more motivated.

An especially effective approach is to combine the gathering of history through a genogram and learning the skills of good communication with a problem-solving approach. If a couple, for example, is constantly fighting over the limits that should be imposed on the children (the children have to finish their homework before dinner versus doing it whenever they want as long as they get it done), you could do a genogram to help the parents see how their families, and hence their expectations and models of parenting and decision making, are different (e.g., mothers decide such issues, or the couple talks it out). You could then help them clean up their communication so that they are less likely to trigger arguments and power struggles that undermine their ability to solve the problem, and lead them through the steps to resolving the problem.

For example, help them brainstorm other outside-the-box approaches for dealing with the kid's homework, encourage them to make compromises rather than just giving in, help them recognize when they are reaching an impasse or falling into a power struggle and need to talk about the problem in the room, or recognize that they need to stop and cool down. By doing all this, you're monitoring the process as it unfolds, can see exactly how and where communication breaks down, and can intervene to help the couple be successful right there in the session. On the heels of such success they are more likely to practice the skills at home, and to see therapy as an effective process.

If you come from a psychodynamic orientation, you view marriage as a process of projective identification in which each partner sees not the real person but rather one disguised with all the unresolved issues from his or her past. Mary sees her husband as harsh and brutally critical just like her father, even though in reality he's not. Or Fred hasn't resolved the desertion of his mother when he was young and spends much of his energy "being good" and repressing most of his anger so that his wife won't get angry and leave him.

Your task becomes one of exploring the past (perhaps with a genogram) and helping the individuals separate past and present issues as well as emotionally resolve unhealed wounds through interpretations or experiences. For example, you may ask Fred to write a letter to his mother expressing how he feels about her abandonment, or have Mary imagine her husband sitting next to her in an empty chair and telling him how she feels when he criticizes her. As the projections are peeled away, the real person can be seen and the overreactions can stop.

Finally, you may want to start your couple assessment with techniques and tools of brief, solution-oriented therapy such as the "Miracle Question." Steve De Shazer and his students always introduce it with an air of mystery and whimsy: "I have a rather strange question. Suppose tonight, while you were asleep, a miracle occurred. When you woke up in the morning you discovered that the problem with . . . Arnold's truancy, your sexual problems, Betty's whining, whatever . . . was miraculously gone! How would it change your relationship?"

Even if you decide not to use a solution-oriented approach (e.g., helping them imagine how they would act if the problem wasn't there), the couple's answer can give you a clue as to the centrality of the problem in their lives, their motivation for changing it, or even the ways things might get worse (e.g., they may admit that they may have nothing to talk about).

Whatever approach you use, however, your choice will be pragmatically overshadowed by the couple's expectations. We're back to the question of who has the problem. For some couples the children have been so much a focus of their attention, either because the couple is child-centered or the children's behavior has created the most problems, that any discussion of their relationship, by you through your questions, or by them through their own initiation, is too fraught with anxiety. The message clearly given is that they are there to help the children and everything else is hands off.

At the other extreme are those couples who drop the subject of children within a few minutes of the first session. When you ask them why they think the presenting problem is happening, they immediately begin their tales of woe and rage about each other. The children, it turns out, were merely the ticket of admission into the therapy system. The focus from the start is upon the relationship.

Again, as mentioned at the beginning of this chapter, some therapists, especially those trained only to work with adults, are quite happy to shift from the children to the marital relationship, never coming back to work on the children issues. This is a mistake on two counts. While it's true that in the long haul children will generally do okay if the couple is doing okay, one or two of the kids may have developed individual problems (e.g., encopresis, extremely aggressive behavior) that need the specific parental and professional attention. To ignore such behaviors or assume that they will automatically get better may result in the children only continuing to do worse, or the couple becoming dragged back into their old patterns. Similarly, even if the problem with the children isn't severe, the couple needs to be able to apply their improved relationship skills to parenting. If they don't, or if you as the therapist aren't sure how well they can, parenting issues may remain the couple's Achilles heel and eventually erode the gains that they have made.

One step back from those couples who declare from the outset that their relationship is the problem, and probably more common, are those cases where an individual parent comes in because of a problem with a child, but then quickly switches focus to the other parent—"I think the kids are having so much trouble these days because me and my wife have just not been getting along." The parent leads the way into the relationship, and you can decide to invite the other parent in, coach the parent on ways of talking at home to his or her spouse about problems, work with the parent individually to increase insight into his or her role in the relationship and problems, help him or her become the change-agent in the family, or offer to help him or her with the child's problems and refer the parent to someone else for individual or couple work. What option you choose again will depend upon your theory and the client's expectations.

In between these positions of staunch resistance and open acceptance of marital problems are the infinite degrees of variation, from the willingness to explore the relationship only as it pertains to the I.P. (child), to the possibility that improving communication may help coordinate parenting, to some agreement that yes, the couple issues probably are affecting the rest of the family and couple therapy might be helpful. Your initial task is to close the gap that lies between your view of the family problems and that of the couple. If you believe that the children and family cannot get better unless this couple gets better, you must persuade them—by education, by underscoring the dysfunctional process in the room, by exploring the ways that emotions spill over to the children, by tracking and highlighting the distortions in the family structure that their relationship engenders. In spite of what they assume, their relationship is not separate from the world of their children. It is the hub onto which everything else in the family holds.

Eric and Cathy, for example, the couple we met at the beginning of this chapter, were by the second session openly acknowledging their divided approach to the children, and the breaking up of the sibling group into father and mother camps. The fact that both were so quickly and openly arguing about it makes it easy for you to talk about their relationship and the struggle they are having not only with the kids, but with each other. They may easily decide that they need to leave the children at home for a few weeks so that they can sort out some of these parenting/ couple issues. The three of you may then decide to bring the children back in and do total family sessions to translate their skills into the parenting structure, or let them do it on their own at home and simply check in with you.

If, however, Eric had refused to talk with Cathy about her concerns, or denied there was any difference in their parenting styles and kept the focus only on the children, you would have had to create a new starting point for discussing the relationship and linking it to the children. You might, for example, have asked Cathy how she felt about Eric's minimizing of her complaints and have wondered aloud if this happens at home as well. Or you may have turned to Eric and asked if he's heard this all before, or if Cathy seems to always find problems where he feels there are none. These questions, this empathizing with each partner's feelings, ideally would encourage the couple to talk about their relationship in a broader way, and help them to talk more openly to each other there in the session.

The process that emerges between them could then be used as a springboard for talking about parenting and the problems the children are having: "I notice that the more impatient you seem, Cathy, to change what the kids are doing, the more, Eric, you say that there's not that much of a problem. I wonder if the kids hear the same thing at home, pick up the split between you both, and wind up playing one of you against the other in order to get their way?"

Of course it's possible to work on the relationship through the family work. Tina and Marcia, for example, a lesbian couple raising two of Tina's children from a previous marriage, came in with the children because of minor behavioral problems with the oldest boy, Tim, age six, at school. Although the couple had been together for several years, it became quickly clear to the therapist that Marcia's role with the children was not clearly and consistently defined. At times Tina would be upset because Marcia would not take an active disciplinary role with the children, while at other times she castigated Marcia for doing precisely that. When the therapist tried to explore the issues of control and decision making between them, both quickly became resistant.

Rather than pressing the issue, the therapist asked the boy to describe his view of the problem, which highlighted for the couple his confusion in knowing who he should turn to for permission. The therapist then asked Tina and Marcia to work up some guidelines that Tim could use in order to clarify communication and ease the boy's confusion. They were both willing to do this.

The next week Tina and Marcia reported just how difficult the process was. Both felt they were engaged in a power struggle. The therapist asked them if they would be willing to use the session to work together and develop guidelines right there and then. By monitoring the process in the room, the therapist helped them recognize when they were starting to get into a power struggle, and by focusing on their communication and encouraging them to compromise, helped them come up with boundaries that both of them could live with. The guidelines they developed, and the negotiation experience itself, laid a foundation not only for helping Tim with his school problems, but for making decisions about the other children as well.

Another therapist might have taken a different path: exploring Tina's unresolved past marital issues, for example: discussing the stresses they felt about being a same-sex couple; examining the children's own response to Tina and Marcia's relationship; or spending play therapy time with the boy to uncover his inner struggles, loss, or adjustment to the family transitions. All these are valid and possible, and may be met with more or less resistance that the therapist would need to negotiate.

Are there times when it would be beneficial for the children to be part of the couple work? Some therapists would say that as soon as the focus shifts to the couple's relationship the children should be out of there; their exclusion helps demarcate for the couple the boundary between couple and parenting issues. If the interaction between the parents is openly hostile and destructive, it's easy for children to feel overwhelmed or blamed (even hearing their name mentioned a lot is enough to cause little kids to think what is happening is their fault). And, of course, if the topics to be discussed are clearly adult topics (e.g., sex, money, adult relationships), if the parents feel inhibited or too easily distracted around the children, or when you feel you can't manage all those people in one room and you can't get a cotherapist, make it easy on everyone and send the children out.

The other side of this issue, however, is that there is value in the children, especially older children, seeing adults communicate and work out problems. The work between the couple may be good modeling for the children of communication and problem solving in relationships, or the process can help the children see the underside of the tension in and between the parents and can come away with a more balanced view of a parent (e.g., Mom isn't just angry all the time, but is worried or sad about Grandma). They can discover or see right before them that they are not to blame for the family's problems, that problems lie elsewhere. With your direct blocking, they can learn that they don't need to step in, take sides, or try to fix what is happening, but can instead let the parents work it out themselves.

Your decision to include children or not ultimately rests on your confidence that the session will be positive, rather than hurtful for the children, that you will not be inadvertently re-creating the dysfunctional structure in the session (pulling in children and triangulating the couple's relationship rather than helping the couple work out their own problems), and that your approach fits both your values and operating theory. Similarly, whatever way you decide to integrate couple work into the family work, it's best that it be integrated both with the other issues in the family and your own view of the system.

What to do about the couple is part of your assessment of what to do about the family and the problem. You don't want to replicate the problem (e.g., ignore the couple issues the way the couple does), or become swept up in the dysfunctional patterns and roles (e.g., giving into the father just like his wife does). Remember, you're in charge of the therapy.

Looking Within: Chapter 13 Exercises

Again the biggest difference between couple and family work isn't the number of people in the room but your own reactions to what the couple presents. These exercises encourage you to become aware of your own professional and personal biases.

1. What is your own theory of couple work? How is it different from and similar to total family work or child therapy? What are your basic assumptions?

2. What are your personal values regarding relationships? What are the limits, if any, of commitments? Where do you draw the line between the couple's problems and the welfare of the children? How open should the couple be with the children about the couple relationship? Who, in what circumstances, has higher priority—the partner, the child, the self? How do you personally decide?

3. If you had siblings while growing up, think back to your relationships. How much sibling rivalry was there in your family? How did your parents handle it? What was the cause or what function do you think it may have served in your family dynamics?

[14]

Couple Repair

S o does couple work seem a bit intimidating? The countertransference seem a little too concentrated? Remind you too much of treating your parents, yourself? The easiest way to think of couple work and stay reasonably objective is to see it as a smaller version of family work. You are still dealing, after all, with patterns and process. Here are the guidelines and goals for family work translated into couple dynamics:

• *Improve communication.* It's hard to overestimate the value of simply getting two people to stay in a room and talk. This is Therapy 101 basics—facilitate the process so that they can learn to take turns, help them talk about themselves rather than just blaming or criticizing the other person, encourage them to talk about their emotions rather than just their ideas and rationalizations, push them to talk about what they haven't talked about before. You can see your job as a coach or traffic cop, a teacher, a role model, or all of the above. Give them communication exercises (have each repeat what he or she thought the other said before saying something else), teach them about "I statements," educate them about the differences between male and female communication styles (e.g., men tend to want to come up with solutions to a problem and be done with it, while their partners are hankering for them to shut up, listen, and discuss the problem together), or try having them communicate nonverbally—sculpting, pictures, clay (the guys will hate it). Most of all, help them experience intimacy by communicating what they have never communicated before.

How much do you need to control the communication between the couple? It depends. As in family therapy, you initially want them to talk to each other so that you can see just how well they can communicate: where things go well, how and where does communication starts to break down, when you have to stop them from trying to direct all their communication through you so they don't become too dependent on you and even more anxious about talking to each other at home. Once you've figured out their communication patterns, you can begin to block and change the patterns ("Hector, you're blaming Teresa and she's feeling scolded and getting defensive. Try telling her how you feel and what you'd like her to do").

Obviously, if their communication is really destructive you will want to take more control over the process and ask them to talk to you rather than the partner, or see them separately in order to decrease the verbal and nonverbal triggers that set the other person off. But as they improve, give them more leeway (you can stare at your shoes when they are communicating well) and enter the conversation only enough to keep them on track and keep the communication open and honest.

There are two common mistakes that therapists make in teaching couples how to communicate better. One is that they don't match their teaching with the couple's expectations. For example, doing formal communication exercises (e.g., starting a series of statements with "I feel . . .") may effectively teach skills, but will be met with resistance if the couple feels emotionally pressured to talk about the argument they had Thursday night, or if the husband sees this as confirming his worst fears about the stupidity of therapy. Wait until the emotional turbulence subsides or connect your exercise to the husband's concern. Your teaching needs to match the couple's needs in terms of timing and content.

A more serious mistake is moving too quickly with angry couples. Your goal is to create success experiences. Couples who cannot yet communicate well or who may intellectually understand good communication skills but haven't practiced them enough yet in their sessions shouldn't be encouraged to discuss topics, especially sensitive ones, at home on their own too soon. Without your protective presence the communication falls apart, the outcome is emotionally or even physically destructive, and their confidence in you and the therapy is broken.

• *Stop violence.* You need to be sensitive to the presence of violence even when the couple doesn't seem to fit your profile of the violent couple, or when they themselves don't bring it up. Ask them matter-of-factly to tell you about their worst argument so you can get some idea of just how bad it can get. Be clear and firm in saying that while emotional or physical violence is a product of other, underlying emotions and problems, as well as their own interaction, they individually need to be responsible for their behavior. Violence has no place in their relationship.

One of the keys to violence prevention is the couple's ability to realize when, in the moment, the argument is crossing over the line and becoming destructive. Often couples can identify the triggers themselves ("We do fine until she starts bringing up things from the past." "I can stay calm until he raises his voice and starts shaking his finger at me." "I'm fine until she says she's done talking and starts to walk out the room"). You, as the outsider, can also identify the verbal and nonverbal triggers in the process of the session; clearly stop and label them so that the couple can begin to do the same. In the beginning it's a good idea to have them "save" arguments from home (e.g., ask them to write down complaints on a list during the week) and have them bring them into the session where you can help them talk them out.

Having them sign a nonviolence contract can help emphasize their self-responsibility, and one of the best techniques is to help them come up with nonverbal signals that either one can use when he or she feels the conversation is getting too hot and needs to stop. Just as it is fruitless for a parent to try and reason with an out-of-control teen, partners trying to reason with the other who is extremely upset is like talking to someone who is psychotic. They need to learn to fix the problem in the room, that is, the escalating emotions, and shift from a verbal to nonverbal medium. (I once saw a "family therapy masters" video where the husband decided he would drop his pants as a signal when conversations were getting out of control. Obviously you can suggest using simpler methods like waving a handkerchief, throwing a kitchen towel in the air, or dropping a book.) Once everyone is cooled off, they can try again to discuss the problem.

If you feel the emotions are just too volatile and the situation is too dangerous, don't be afraid to recommend that the couple temporarily separate until they and you can get things under control. Again, you want change and success, not replication and failure. Once you've helped the couple stop falling into the violent patterns, you can begin to focus on the underlying issues and emotions generating the anger.

• *Educate them about emotions and relationships.* I often see couples where one partner is identified as having an "anger problem." The angry partner often seeks therapy because he or she is desperate to "get straightened out." The long-suffering victim is finally fed up and has threatened to leave or has actually walked out of the relationship. My goals with the angry partner are to help him or her increase emotional range so that anger is not the only expression for myriad more subtle emotions, learn to recognize the onset of strong emotions (such clients often emotionally go from zero to 60 in nanoseconds and are unaware of the earlier emotional cues), and solve the chronic problems that keep the couple in continual turmoil.

For a good number of these individuals, I've found, there is a history of childhood emotional and often physical abuse. Their quick, angry overreactions are actually the hypervigilance of posttraumatic stress disorder. Their anger is a self-sufficient "me against the world" stance, a learned means of coping and protecting themselves against what seems to them to be a constantly threatening and frightening environment. If this is the case (ask about their childhoods—if they say their parents were "strict," explore further), they often need help understanding the source of their overreaction, help talking about the underlying pain that drives the anger, help separating out the past from the present, coaching to help them substitute assertiveness for anger (i.e., adopting an adult response rather than continuing that of the frightened child), and encouragement to attempt active experiments in trust.

The goal with the other partner is to move beyond the aggressor–victim scenario he or she has overidentified with and mentally clings to. The partner needs to see how he or she unwittingly feeds into the destructive pattern, and like the spouse, struggles with assertiveness. This makes the problem more balanced. It is no longer one person as the aggressor, the other the victim. Both are responsible for changing the patterns; both need to learn self-responsibility and self-regulation.

For all couples it's always useful to help them realize that though their emotional styles may be different, they are both feeling exactly the same: "It seems from what you both have described that you both are feeling ignored and lonely, but you express it differently. Liz, you seem to get quiet and withdraw, while your style, Matt, is to get irritable and demanding. What you naturally react to, of course, is the withdrawal or demands, but underneath you both are feeling the same." In contrast to the differences that they are only too aware of, you are helping them see commonalities.

Finally, educate them about normal developmental change. Ask the couple what each of them needed most when they got married or met. Looking back, how were they different people then than the way they are now? How did the partner help fill those earlier needs? Then ask them to talk what they need now, for themselves, from the relationship.

You can then weave these answers together, highlighting that they're both saying that they've changed over the years, that what they needed at the beginning they no longer need now because they have each grown, in part due to the help of their partner. But the current needs and current people don't fit within the box that the marriage has become with its set patterns and silent rules, and so they complain, blame, or argue, or have fantasies of getting divorced or having affairs. "What you are experiencing is something that happens in most couples after six, seven, eight years of marriage." Having a developmental context for their struggle helps them feel less guilty or overwhelmed. The real goal is to create a new vision of the relationship that better represents who they are today.[1]

- *Help them recognize when and how the children are a solution/distraction.* As mentioned several times earlier, you need to help the couple see the link between the children's problems and their relationship. Specifically, you want to help them see how and when the children are being triangled into the relationship, and the way the children's problems can become distractions from their own. This point of view in effect makes the children's problems barometers of the couple relationship. When the kids start arguing more than they were, when Tommy's grades start dropping off once again, it's a signal not only that they need to intervene together to help the children, but that they need to look at something that they may need to be worked out in their relationship.[2]

- *Teach problem-solving skills.* While most couples will come in with a handful of problems that they need help resolving, your job isn't so much helping them solve them as teaching them the skills they need to solve those and other problems that will come along in the future. Good problem solving involves good communication, a realistic view of the way re-

---

[1]One of the books that I've found useful when working with couples is Harville Hendrix, *Getting the Love You Want*, Owl Books, 2001. He includes 10 exercises, including one on helping couples create a new vision of their relationship that you can assign as homework.

[2]Another good, client-friendly book for couples on system dynamics and triangulation is Maggie Scarf, *Intimate Partners*, Ballantine, 1988.

lationships work, and the ability for both partners to be clear and assertive about their needs and to know what the problem really is.

So as you help the couple work through the problems and arguments they bring to the session, identify the skills ("You both did a good job talking about your feelings"), help them generalize the process ("You both were able to talk about Jane without getting angry. What did you both do that made it easier this time?"), and assist them in getting over communication hurdles ("Bill, you seem to be just passively going along with what Lynn says. I wonder if you are reluctant to disagree. What do you, yourself, really want here?"). Look at your role as more of a coach fine-tuning what they present, rather than a lecturer merely dumping out a lot of information. Instead of getting wrapped up in the content of a problem, help them recognize good problem-solving process.

• *Sensitize them to their power issues.* It's not only violent couples who need to be able to tell when problem solving turns into power struggling, when who makes the decision or who gets the last word has become more important than what the decision or word is. All couples need to be able to recognize when discussions are escalating, know what topics are potential land mines for them ("We realize that we can't talk about my mother, your drinking, the affair I had two years ago"), recognize when these topics are being used as ammunition in arguments, and be able to stop before things get out of hand. You as the therapist and outsider are the one to set the pace on this. You are often the first to clarify the process and point out the emotions that accompany the power struggle.

• *Create a united front/support the underdog.* Not only is there the selling of the idea of working together, but helping the couple make the transition and do it. Sometimes therapists make the mistake of not adequately mapping out with the couple exactly the behavioral changes they need to make at home. Their anxiety and uncertainty causes the couple to fall back into their old patterns and leaves the therapist erroneously believing that they are being resistant.

If Ms. Smith, for example, has always left the discipline to her husband, or has taken sides with the children, her shift to a stronger role will be a difficult one. Help her say what support she needs from her spouse ("I need you to tell me that I've done a good job"; "I need you to literally stand next to me when I tell the kids to go to bed"; "I need you to tell Rachel to ask me if she can go out to play") in order to help her avoid becoming overwhelmed by the children, in order to give him a new role and task, in order to help them both avoid easily slipping back into the old patterns. Whatever strategy is developed, it needs to be specific and well planned ahead of time.

• *Create positive interactions.* Affection anyone? How about a night out without the kids? As you help push the children back into their appropriate roles, as you cool down the conflict, something needs to fill the space or it will just fill back up again. Couples who have gone for years living with distance, children as buffers, and conflict instead of positive interaction need not only to learn to stop what they are doing, but gradually to learn to feel comfortable with intimacy and support.

Pacing is the key here and it's important not to move too quickly. The couple that hasn't been out on a date for 10 years is going to have an anxious time when they do. They could easily wind up talking the entire time about what Johnny did wrong this week, or arguing about whether the restaurant is too expensive.

You can begin by increasing intimacy and risk within the session— helping them to talk about each other rather than the children, about what they like rather than what they don't. You can help them plan together some small exercise in quality time (watch a video together after the kids go to bed that they want to see, rather than always watching kid movies) and normalize the anxiety they may feel. Again you need to be sensitive and walk that fine line between approaching their anxiety, and opening up communication and intimacy (go ahead, casually ask them about their sex lives), and scaring them and causing them to back away (okay, maybe that wasn't a good idea—go back and ask them how they feel about your bringing up sexual issues). As they get more positive experience with each other, and you, they'll be able to move on to bigger activities and challenges.

• *Block the patterns.* The couple work is like the family work. Stop the dysfunctional patterns and see what happens.

STEPPING INTO THE QUAGMIRE

Yes, the couple work isn't much different from the family work, but it can seem more difficult for several reasons. By seeing the couple alone you are by definition creating another awkward triangle. Instead of the children, it's you who's in the middle, and like them you may feel tempted to form

coalitions, to be a buffer or distraction between them, or not take sides so
no one gets mad at you. As with family work with children, the easiest
way to avoid the tension of such triangles is to define them as they arise,
in the room and in the process, in order to keep the focus on the couple
and their anxiety.

Balance is essential in couple work. If you decide to see one partner
separately, be sure to see the other separately as well. If you talk with one
about goals, talk to the other about goals too. Leaving things off-balance
is dangerous. Spending more time with one partner than the other fuels
fears that you are both ganging up, forming a more intimate relationship,
or that you really believe that the other person is the one with all the
problems and most in need of your attention. It stirs old sibling rivalry
feelings. Be clear about your treatment decisions and sensitive to possible
misinterpretation.

But before you step into the room you need to be sensitive to yourself
as well. You may be seduced into playing out a role, identifying with one
side over another not only because of the parent's needs and patterns, but
yours. How you are doing or not doing in your own relationships can easily color what you see before in the room.

If, for example, you've just been arguing with your husband about his
doing more work around the house, or his taking off every Saturday to
play golf or watch football with the guys, you may find yourself identifying
with the woman across from you who complains that her husband
"doesn't do a damn thing except sit in front of the TV," or with the husband who says he hates the way his wife stays on the phone talking to her
family for what seems like 12 hours a day. It's tempting to use their process
to express vicariously your depression, your loneliness, your anger—
"Doesn't that make you angry, Helen? Why don't you tell Alan just how
angry you feel." Who's getting therapy here? With rationalizations you
may even encourage the couple to play out your own desire for a divorce.

The subtlety of this countertransference–transference process is even
more enhanced if you choose to see the partners individually. The man
who flirts as a way of coping with his anxiety may successfully re-create
with you the affair he has had, is having, or that he and you fantasize
about. The woman who "just would like to meet with you alone next time
to discuss some personal issues" may help to create the friendship, the intimacy that she, and you, don't have in your current relationships. Each
person becomes a blank screen for the other's fantasies and projections.

The solution, of course, is awareness, asking yourself the hard questions: What do I need from my personal relationship that I'm not getting? What do I need most from my clients? How can I tell when I'm overidentifying with a client, when I'm encouraging them to do what I have trouble doing myself? It also helps to have people around (e.g., supervisors; trusted, experienced colleagues; your own therapist) who will help you practice what you preach and separate your personal issues from professional ones.

LONG-DISTANCE FEUDS

Mark comes in to see you with his 10-year-old daughter, Maggie, of whom he has custody. He describes Maggie as "wild and disrespectful" for three or four days after her visits with her mother two weekends a month. He also thinks he knows what the problem is, namely, that his ex just "lets Maggie do anything she wants, and basically neglects her." He says he wants help in managing Maggie after these visits, and by the way, he's thinking of going back to court to stop the visitations all together. He wonders aloud whether you would at some point consider writing a letter giving your professional opinion about this.

Just as there are infinite points along the continuum regarding the ability of the couple in the home to own their relationship problems, the same continuum can be found in long-distance conflictual relationships between separated or divorced partners and parents. Doing couple work where there is no couple, where the child is still triangled and caught in a cross-fire between two warring parents is not uncommon, and not easy.

Just as the couple or ex-couple is blurring the lines between themselves and their pasts, and themselves and their children, it can become easy for your role to blur as well. The best defense in these cases is a good offense, namely, defining for yourself and the client as quickly and clearly as possible just what you will and will not do, what you see as appropriate goals and what are not, what is considered therapeutic and what is a legal matter. In order not to get sucked in you need to do what this couple apparently cannot.

With Mark, for example, it would be important to clarify exactly what he needs help with in relation to Maggie. Is he asking for management techniques or an expectation that you will see Maggie alone to help her work out her tumultuous emotions following the visits? Is he asking for a formal evaluation of Maggie for court testimony or is there an unspoken expectation that through your individual contacts with Maggie you will gather information from her that he can then subpoena to use in court? If your client seems to be trying to corner you into making a legal recommendation, don't hesitate to suggest that the client contact his or her attorney about this, or request that the attorney make a formal request. Make it clear, get it out on the table; be sure once again that you know who has and what is the problem, and who is your client.

If your initial impression is that the problem is less the child than the ongoing battle between the parents, you can say this. The next step is then to invite the absent parent in and help the parents work together. This may involve helping to come up with some mutually agreed ways of managing the child (e.g., both agree to enforce the same bedtimes), move deeper and help them resolve their continuing issues, or farm the whole thing out to trained mediators or other marital therapists. By having both parents in front of you, you avoid getting sucked in and triangled into an ongoing battle between the parents.

Some therapists will refuse to see the case unless they can actually see both parents together; others don't necessarily have to see them in the office, but want to have at least telephone contact with the other parent (for example, when the other parent lives out-of-state) so that they can hear both sides of the story, clarify what the child may need and encourage the parents to work together. Again the goal is to avoid taking sides and replicating the triangle that already exists with the child.

Of course, you have some responsibility to advocate for the child if you feel that there is reason for worry. If, for example, you learn from Maggie that she is being neglected or being placed in unsafe situations, if she talks about potential or real emotional, physical, or sexual abuse situations, you have a responsibility to notify the proper authorities, usually social services, so that they can pursue a formal investigation. There may be times where there is a fine line between your sense of what may be happening to the child and what the child may feel pressure to report by the parent. If the parent reports to you that he or she thinks the child is being abused or neglected, but you have no first-hand evidence yourself, you may want to contact your local protective services to clarify their protocols and tell the parent to make a formal report as well.

If you have any doubt (and in cases like this there may often be doubt), contacting the proper authorities (and your supervisor, if appropriate) is the best approach. They have the mandate to do the investigation and your role as therapist, rather than investigator, stays clear.

As with other couple work, these long-distance conflicts have a way of emotionally pulling you in, particularly if you have similar unresolved issues yourself. Hearing only one side of the story, seeing the poor child caught in the middle, it's easy to emotionally join the bandwagon against one or both of the parents, easy to overidentify with the child.

Clarity is the antidote—with the client, with yourself through self-reflection and supervision. Bring someone else to work the case with you, have someone else see the child, have a team behind the mirror observe the session process, gather court records to find out if there is a court order and legal mandates, talk to the guardian ad litem and clarify roles and gather background. Do what you need to do to prevent yourself from becoming swept up in already emotionally sweeping family dynamics.[3]

COUPLES AND CONTEXT

Parents share two relationships—the one as caretakers of their children, the other, their relationship as a couple. While they often enter therapy with the line between these relationships blurred, or with their focus only on one and not the other, your job is to help them distinguish between both relationships, as well as show how each is connected.

As has been said throughout this chapter, this clarity is important in order for the family to remain structurally and emotionally healthy. It's hard enough being a child without having to get dragged into acting like an adult or taking the blame for problems that the adults aren't handling. It's easy, but detrimental, as a parent to turn to your children for support or distraction when you feel overwhelmed or overlooked in your relationship with your partner.

Because the couple's relationship is made of the same basic building blocks of patterns and process as the family's, your other family skills will serve you as you begin work with them. Keep in mind the basics, don't be afraid to move against their grain and yours, and, once again, above all be honest.

---

[3]There are a number of texts on marital therapy that are useful: Philip Guerin, *The Evaluation and Treatment of Marital Conflict*, Basic Books, 1987; William Nichols, *Marital Therapy: An Integrative Approach*, Guilford Press, 1988; Peter Martin, *A Marital Therapy Manual*, Jason Aronson, 1994; Alan Gurman, *Casebook of Marital Therapy*, Guilford Press, 1991.

Looking Within: Chapter 14 Exercises

1. What did you learn from your parents about the nature of relationships? How has their relationship shaped your expectations of your own? What did you learn about how problems in the relationship should be solved? What mistake(s) did your parents make that you would most like to avoid?

2. Think about your current or past intimate relationships. What issues most trigger your anger, the urge to leave? What topics easily most easily turn into power struggles or impasses? Why?

3. How do you personally define intimacy? What role does or did sex play in your current or past relationships? How do any of these issues create countertransference problems for you when doing couples therapy?

[15]

The Power of One

INDIVIDUAL WORK
IN A FAMILY CONTEXT

Ann talks with a slow whine, each word barely limping ahead of the one before. She looks drained, and she tells you how she spends hours in the middle of the night pacing up and down, just sitting at the kitchen table, or lying in bed staring up at the darkness. To her everything seems gray; even things that used to excite her—an evening with friends, a new project at work—seem now like another burden, another responsibility. She sighs, one of those long, heavy sighs that stretches out and fills the room.

Major depression? Dysthymia? Adjustment disorder with depression? Bereavement? Whatever you call it, it has DSM-IV written all over it. Individual therapy here we come.

But if you're a family therapist, you may feel, or think you ought to feel, uncomfortable with this. Not only is the room a bit too empty, but you feel a flutter of hesitation at the thought of plodding into that swamp of individual pathology and internal dynamics.

Don't fear. In this chapter we explore together how to work with individuals and still consider yourself a family therapist. Family therapy, after all, isn't about how many people you can cram into a room, but about how many people you can keep in your mind. It's less about what you do and more about how you think—looking at problems and people in terms of their patterns and interactions. With this perspective you can help others change one person or help one person change others. They're really both sides of the same fence.

IS IT ME?

But most clients don't look at their problems in this interactive way; from where they sit the problem and the coin only has one side. In an agency or clinic setting someone like Ann may call up, come in by herself, and be seen by someone in intake who notes on the intake form "probable depression." When she shows up alone in your office she will talk about their problems as being caused by herself ("I am the problem") or by others ("My mother is the problem"). Whatever way clients may present their problem doesn't really matter. What's important is that you offer them a perspective that they don't have.

We're talking again about giving the client a different theory and problem to replace one that has become too familiar and comfortable, about seeing what's missing and moving toward their anxiety. If Ann, for example, only talks about all the awful things she feels she did in the past, goes on and on about the way her husband is always screwing up her life, or laments about her mother who never really cared about her, she's not wrong in her view, simply stuck within it. You will need to start by hearing and acknowledging her perspective, but then you want to encourage her to look at the other side of the coin and focus on what she's not seeing.

If she is only talking about the past, you want to know about the present. Instead of blaming her husband or mother, you want to help her draw lines of responsibility between herself and them, as well as see her own role in the interactions. By helping Ann recognize what she can and can't control, by encouraging her to talk in new ways about new topics, you are helping her mobilize her energy and resources in a new and potentially more positive direction.

You also want to introduce the client to systemic thinking and the power of patterns by asking about them: "So what does your mother say when you tell her how you feel?" "What do you say back?" "How do these conversations usually wind up?" Questions like these can help the clients begin to recognize that there is an interactional dynamic at work shaping their problems and emotions; they may come to see their past decisions in a less self-accusatory, black–white way. By helping Ann, for example, see how her mother and husband are individuals influenced by their own psychological networks of others may not excuse their actions, but can cast them as less villainous and more human. By sidestepping blame and guilt, by developing a more complete view of her relationships and problems, Ann can gain a greater sense of mastery, which in turn can serve as an antidote to depression.

The answer then to the question "Is the problem me?" is "Yes, at least in part, if you don't think it is," and "No, maybe not," if you feel absolutely sure that it is. The goal is not to identify the culprits but expand thinking beyond either/or dichotomies. You are not the victim or the persecutor, but often both and neither; you affect and are affected by those around you.

COME ON IN: USING THE FAMILY TO HELP THE INDIVIDUAL

If you believe that problems are interactional, then it makes sense to bring in all those individuals who interact and intersect around a problem—this, of course, the tried and true basis of family therapy. But even if you or the client decide that switching from individual to some form of ongoing family therapy isn't reasonable, there are still plenty of ways to enlist the help of important others.

One is to bring in significant others for one or two information-gathering sessions. For example, when Cassandra talked about her guilt over the abusive way she felt she had treated her sister when they were teenagers, the therapist suggested that she invite her sister to one of their sessions. She did, and Cassandra spent the time in a monologue, delivered with much hesitation and anxiety, about the way she felt about those times past. Cassandra had the opportunity to say what she could not say, to put into words what she had only grieved inside for years. The proclamation, the confession, was itself therapeutic.

Having the right audience made it even more so. Her sister did what often happens in such situations. She acknowledged what Cassandra had said—how she had felt both hurt and confused by Cassandra's behavior, how her memories of that time continued to strain their relationship in the present—but then she turned the corner and talked about her own regret and guilt. She apologized for not understanding how hard their parents had been on her, for walling her off over the years, and most of all for failing to show her appreciation for all that Cassandra had done for her— Cassandra's offer, for example, to take her in when she was having a difficult time in college, her reaching out with consolation and support when her daughter had died several years before.

Healing occurred because Cassandra not only repented and was forgiven, but because the distorted memories were corrected. She discovered through her sister a new way of viewing herself and her actions that would have been difficult to achieve without the feedback of this family member.

Other times the focus such sessions is less on healing of the past and more on solving a problem in the present. Louis had just started dating Nadine, but he was already struggling with what he thought were her expectations over how much time they should spend together. Because the relationship was still new, Louis didn't feel comfortable starting any ongoing couple therapy. He did, however, agree that it might be helpful to have Nadine come to one of his individual therapy sessions just to discuss the topic.

She came in the next session, and the dialogue enabled Louis to deal with his feelings and concerns in a much more direct way than he had in the past. Rather than remaining silent and ruminating, he was able to be assertive in the session; rather than assuming he knew what Nadine wanted, he took the risk to ask her. Nadine came away with an honest picture of the kind person Louis was, and he had the opportunity to start a new relationship with a different set of patterns.

Sometimes the motivation of having others come into individual therapy is more yours than the client's. Individual therapy is by definition limited in its view. You as the therapist may want others to come in to provide a more complete and accurate picture of the past or present, or to help you better grasp the interactional patterns that have occurred or are ongoing.

Those that you invite in essentially serve as consultants. Rather than using the session as a forum for solving problems or disclosing long-held secrets, the focus is upon uncovering the important information you feel is missing. The client listens, and in the listening can step back and perhaps hear what couldn't be heard before.

For example, in the course of her individual treatment, Molly talked about the ways she felt favored by her alcoholic father, while he seemed to ignore her other brothers and sisters. The therapist asked if she would invite her brother, who lived in town, to come with her for a session. He did, and in contrast to Cassandra's session with her sister, it was the therapist who asked questions of the brother. She asked how he viewed his father's relationship with Molly and the other children, and what sense he had made out of his childhood years.

Not only did the therapist gain a different and more rounded view of the early family life, but Molly, sitting quietly in the corner, heard reactions and feelings and answers to questions that, because of her own blind spots, anxiety, and assumptions, she would never have been aware of. Because the session focus and process wasn't on her, she was able to really hear what her brother was saying, and, like Cassandra, was offered a new vision of her past.

While bringing others into individual therapy is clearly a good way of reshaping the past and present, such sessions need to be carefully planned. The guests need to know why they're there. They're undoubtedly anxious about what might happen and may have all kinds of fantasies about the session turning into an interrogation or trial. They need to be welcomed, and, either before the session or at its start, need to know exactly what you are planning. Make clear to them that they have a choice—to talk or not to talk, to stop, to ask questions. By being both respectful and in command you can offset their fear that the session will turn into an emotional free-for-all.

You also want to be in charge in order to support your client. Because you don't really know the guests, you don't know what they may or may not say. Cassandra's sister, for example, might have tried to dominate the session from the moment the she sat down, or broken into an angry rant by emotional triggers unknown to you. While getting things out in the open and working through the process are all valuable, no one should wind up at the end of the session feeling emotionally trampled.

One way to ensure that this doesn't happen is to leave sufficient time and space for debriefing and closure. Cassandra shouldn't just deliver her monologue and leave; Louis shouldn't just say what he wants to without hearing what Nadine expects; Molly's brother shouldn't just open his own emotional can of worms and then be thanked for coming. Leave time at the end of the session for wrapping up, discussing the process itself, supporting risk taking. Offer to have the people come back again if necessary.

You need to judge whether your client is ready to handle a live confrontation or confession. Does he or she really think it is a good idea, or is the client merely trying to please you by going along with what he or she thinks you want? Is there any danger that you are unwittingly replicating a problem and dynamic that your client cannot yet emotionally handle or change?

Be honest with yourself whether bringing in others is your way of coping with your anxiety or sloughing off your responsibility. Just like the college professor who fills a course with guest speakers as a way of not having to actually teach the class by him- or herself, you can fill therapy sessions with all kinds of significant others who seem to do the therapy work you yourself should be doing. If you are bringing someone into the session because you don't know what else to do, or are hoping to dissipate the anxiety that the intimacy of individual therapy can create, you're serving your purposes, not the client's. Be clear about your goal and the effect you would like to create, then plan your sessions accordingly. Be clear about whose problem you're trying to solve.

IN LOCO FAMILIA

When family members can't or won't come in—they think therapy is only for crazy people—they often will if the therapist is convinced that it's important. Making the effort to reach out and personally invite the family members, letting them know that their contributions are valuable, and reassuring them that it will not be an interrogation or free-for-all is often enough to get them to participate. Even for family members who live far away, a conference phone call, though not ideal, may be just as useful.

If they refuse and really won't come in, there's always the opportunity to reach out and communicate long distance. You can suggest to your client Ned that he call up and talk to his brother about how disappointed he was that his brother didn't come to his son's wedding, or encourage Alice to write a letter and mail it to her boyfriend, putting into words what she would have said if he could have been there in the session. Such long-distance methods are often easier for the client than the face-to-face meeting. The client may feel less intimidated and less on the spot: Ned can write down what he wants to say before he makes the call; Alice can shape the words in a letter with more consideration.

Your job is to counteract the limitations of the media—the absence of nonverbal feedback, the one-sidedness of the letter. Encourage the client to talk or write completely, that is, to make sure he says not only what he wants the other person to know, but also explains why he is saying it, anticipating the other's possible questions or reactions and building the person's response into the planned phone conversation or letter.

As an example, here is as letter that one woman wrote to her father who was dying of cancer:

Dear Dad,

I've wanted to come see you and I'm sorry that I haven't been able to do so. I hope to come at the end of the month.

I've wanted to write to you for some time because I guess I need to get some things off my chest. When I look back on my teenage years, those early years of my marriage, I still get filled with anger and regret—anger that you left, regret that you weren't part of my life for so long. For a long time I blamed myself, blamed Mom. Much of the trouble I got into, some of the bad decisions that I made I thought would have never happened if you had stayed.

Slowly I'm beginning to see that you didn't leave because of me but because of you and Mom. I wish we hadn't lost that time.

This is a pretty clear letter, but she needed to talk more fully so that her father could better understand why she was saying what she was. Here is the revised letter that she wrote after she and I talked more about her feelings about her father and what she hoped the letter could convey:

Dear Dad,

I've wanted to come and see you and I'm sorry that I haven't been able to do so. I hope to come at the end of the month.

I've wanted to write to you for some time because I guess I need to get some things off my chest. I've been doing a lot of thinking lately about some of the decisions I've made, about my time growing up, trying to understand my past better so that I don't make the same mistakes in the future.

When I look back on my teenage years and those early years of my marriage, I still get filled with anger and regret—anger that you left, regret that you weren't part of my life for so long. For long time I blamed myself, blamed Mom for your leaving. I used to think that somehow you were the reason I got into so much trouble, the reason I made some bad decisions. If only you had stayed, my life, I believed, would have turned out so much different.

And maybe it would have, but I also know that I need to take some responsibility for the life I've led. Finally now I'm beginning to realize that you didn't leave because of me, but because of you and Mom.

It's taken me a long time to figure this out. I'm not writing to make you feel guilty or to hit you over the head with the past. I know you've got your own regrets. I just want to let you know that I'm sorry I've pushed you away for so many years when you did try to come back in my life. I'm sorry that we lost that time between us. I just want to let you know that I love you.

When connections with family are not possible, others can step in to facilitate the change process. Both the systemic notion of interactional patterns and the concept of transference tell us that while people are unique, our relationships with them are not. Each of us re-creates over and over again the same patterns across relationships. By changing the patterns between friends, coworkers, bosses, even strangers, these changes can flow out to change other family members, and flow in to change the client.

This, of course, is the basis of group therapy, where the group members project on each other unresolved emotions and re-create the dynamics of their past relationships. Over time the group becomes a surrogate family. As the interactions are played out, challenged, and changed within the group process, so too are the individual's cognitive and emotional responses that held the patterns in place.

When formal group therapy isn't possible, you can create a mini-group. Have friends, roommates, coworkers, cousins—anybody whom the client feels comfortable inviting—come into session with him or her. By focusing on the process, rather than the content, by looking for replication of patterns (the way John is just as unassertive with his roommate as he is with his sister; the way Cynthia holds back how she feels when her friend hurts her feelings, just as she does when her mother does the same) you are tacking the same problems from a different angle.

Again you need to be clear—about the expectations and goals for the session or sessions, about confidentiality, about the role of the guest. You need to be in charge, be sensitive to the process, and leave time to debrief so that there are not any loose emotional ends left dangling.

Finally, there are cases where neither family nor family surrogates are available. How else can you expand the client's perspective to include the viewpoint of others and create individual change? Some change will naturally come about from your relationship with the client, through your tracking of client's transference, as he or she projects on you significant others from his or her past.

But it's also possible to expand the client's perspective by bringing others in through the client's imagination. Use experiential techniques: letter writing to those who are deceased, complete with their expected or ideal response back to the client; empty chair work—having the client role play both sides of a dialogue between him- or herself and another person from the past or present; guided imagery—helping the client imagine a conversation between him- or herself and an old mentor, the dialogue the client wishes he or she had the last time the client saw Mother, or imagining one's life as a play, with different periods of time (childhood, adolescence, early marriage) as specific scenes on a stage. These techniques and any others that you can create increase your understanding of the client's inner and outer world and expand the therapeutic ground that you both have to work upon. Through the experiential process you are providing opportunities for catharsis, closure, and healing to take place.

THE FIFTH COLUMN

Frank comes to see you, saying that he wants his wife Suzanne to stop crabbing at him all the time. At her first appointment Jane states that she wants to get her 14-year-old son, Paul, to stop talking back to her and to come home on time. Tamisha complains endlessly, it seems, about the way her mother stirs guilt in her every time she calls. She wants her mother to just stop doing it. What do you say to these people?

You can tell them that they need to bring these others into the sessions, that you need to see them to help them change. You may coach them on how to talk to the others about coming in, or you may offer to call the other persons up and invite them in, but you are clear that changing family interactions requires that you see the family.

You can also help them solve their problems by coaching them on ways to change their behaviors at home. The systemic way of thinking says that if Frank changes what he does, Suzanne *must* do the same; as old patterns are broken, new ones will take their place. This is what Billy's grandmother and Ellen's mother, Ms. Harris, were doing as parents—

changing their parenting approach in order to effect change in the children. But this can apply to any relationship within a family. You as the therapist can coach the client to become the change-agent within the family.

Essentially, what you do is teach the individual how to think systemically. Patterns of interactions are tracked down and mapped out, and strategies are developed specifically to change the patterns: "So, Frank, what would happen if you didn't snap back when your wife starts complaining?"; "Tamisha, when your mother calls on Sunday and starts her usual spiel that makes you feel guilty and angry, try telling her how you feel, rather than staying quiet or trying to change the topic"; "Jane, if Paul doesn't come in on time Saturday night, what do you want to do about it? What kinds of consequences can you set that are different than what you have done before?"

"Different than what you have done before" is the key to changing the patterns. Just as you would do in a session, you're pushing the individual to go against the grain, to do something that stirs his or her anxiety, which in turn will stir the anxiety in the other. In order to help the client sustain the change you must think ahead and help anticipate what he or she can do in the face of the other's resistance and opposition—help Frank envision how Suzanne may react, help him decide what he can do when she becomes even more irritable or angry; what Tamisha can say if her mother switches roles and begins to sound guilty herself; what Jane can do when Paul blows up or ignores her when she says he's grounded the next two days.

This type of change making is a slower process than total family or couple work because you're only able to work with one side of the interaction. Your primary job is helping your client to stay the course, especially in the beginning, as the other escalates as a way to quell his or her own anxieties, attempting to push the client back to the old patterns and role ("It gets worse before it gets better"). Predicting the opposition, framing it as the beginning of change, and helping the client know specifically and behaviorally how to respond are essential.

But there is also the challenge of maintaining a new stance over the long haul when increased stress can cause all of the family members to waver and fall back. Frank or Tamisha or Jane may, with job pressures or illness, collapse back to their old responses during those fragile transition times when new patterns have been planted but not yet firmly taken root.

Just as the individual needs to hold a clear vision of what he or she wants and stay committed to it in the face of the resistance, you need to hold a clear vision of what your role and task are. When the client starts to waver, you need to make sure you don't.

INDIVIDUAL DANGERS

This one-person approach to problems and family change can start to sound pretty simple, too simple perhaps—give me any problem, any individual, and I, as the therapist, can coach him or her into getting what he or she wants. Yes and no. Yes, you can help stimulate change by helping your client change, but no, you and the client can't absolutely direct its outcome in others.

But the bigger issue is that there is a bigger issue. The goal isn't only to change patterns and behaviors in another person, but to create change in a relationship for a purpose and to help the other person fully understand what that purpose is. Beyond the changing of patterns is the need to move toward honesty and intimacy. At some point Frank doesn't need only to stop overreacting to Suzanne, he needs to be clear with her about what he wants, what he needs from her and the relationship so that she can do the same. At some point Tamisha must not only teach her mother not to trigger her guilt, but leave enough room in the conversation to tell her mother how she needs her. At some point Jane needs to ask herself why Paul seems so angry at her and how she and he can have a better relationship.

Without this honesty, this bare-bones declaration of who and what is really needed, and wanted, and, most important, without strategies for stopping, dysfunctional patterns become nothing more than a new way of sidestepping in order to keep the other person off balance; the individual may feel more in control, but without self-responsibility, commitment to the relationship, and caring for the other person, he or she is merely being manipulative. The shifting of patterns merely becomes another form of a dysfunctional interaction.

You job is to help the client form this larger picture and take this risk of intimacy. To do this you need to be alert and honest about your therapeutic relationship with the client. Just as couple work becomes more difficult than total family work because the couple's issues can more easily tap into your own personal weak spots, individual work often creates an intimacy that can make the therapeutic relationship more important than the change you're trying to establish. Rather than helping Frank look at what he needs from Suzanne, there's the danger that Frank and his therapist will join forces in seeing her as a problem. Rather than helping Jane expand her relationship with Paul, the therapist and she may spend session after session spinning around the problem so that they have a reason to keep their relationship the same. At some point the therapeutic relationship, while seemingly working to change family patterns, becomes inadvertently another way of replicating them.

These powerful countertransference forces are what make individual therapy so different from other formats. Just as bringing people into the therapy can become a crutch for the therapist to avoid the anxiety of doing the therapy, excluding people can be the rationalized trap for getting your intimacy needs met through your clients.

And if the potential intimacy isn't enough of a seduction, power can be. The dependency of the individual client on the therapist, even when the therapist is helping the individual to change his or her relationships, can be strong, and stronger still can be the therapist's need for the dependency. Again, it's not that this collusion can't happen in other formats, because it can; it's the subtle way the process can be so easily distorted through the narrower, less-distracted focus of the individual therapy. Even though the goal may be problem solving, the problems somehow never seem to end; the dependency may be recognized, but it is rationalized as a necessary step to further future growth.

The fact that the danger is there doesn't mean that individual therapy isn't valuable, or even an approach of choice in its own right. What it does mean is that you need to be curious about the different qualities of your therapeutic relationships, question inconsistencies in your approach, be willing to use supervision to challenge your decisions and plans. If you can, the dangers can be avoided and once again you can serve as a model of honesty and clarity.

BACK TO ANN

So where does all this take us in regard to Ann? Here are some possible therapeutic options to help her with her depression:

- Bring in family members to solve the problems that she's having difficulty solving; to increase their support; to help her be more assertive, more powerful within her relationships; to educate them about depression, to discourage whatever blame or guilt they may be heaping on her.

- If she is relatively isolated, explore dormant family relationships—the sister "who is too busy with her own life to care," the aunt that she's been long out of touch with.

- Bring in nonfamily members or have her start in a therapy group to increase support around her, to develop her social skills, to help her unravel and change the patterns that undermine her power, maintain her stress, compromise her decision-making and problem-solving ability.

- See her individually to help her see how she can change, rather than being victimized by the forces and people around her. Coach her on changing interactional patterns, help her draw clear lines of responsibility around her problem and those of others, between what she can change and what she cannot. Serve as morale booster, an emotional cheerleader for promoting change in her life patterns.

- Refer her for antidepressant medication, coordinate services with the physician, monitor the results along with the physician; be responsible and see if there's a needs for more intensive services, for example, hospitalization or increased supervision. Once she is stable, negotiate with her about her goals and needs for further therapy.

- See her individually to help her learn to apply cognitive-behavioral principles. By helping her track her self-talk ("I always screw up; it's never going to get any better"; "I'm just a basket case") and change the statements ("I'm having a hard time, but I can get help to solve this problem"), she can alter the emotions these statements and this language creates. Teach problem-solving skills and encourage her to be proactive rather than reactive.

- See her individually to resolve issues with people from her past and present; use the support of the therapeutic relationship to help her experiment with risk taking and assertiveness in order to increase her self-confidence; help her increase her emotional awareness and emotional range, especially of strong emotions like anger.

All these and probably more are possible paths to take. The choice once again depends upon the severity of the symptoms, Ann's stated goals, her perception of her problem, her expectations of therapy, as well as your own framework for viewing the problem—your values, comfort, and skills with various approaches, options, and formats. Once you decide on a particular approach, try it and see what happens.

If your plan doesn't seem to be working for her, don't be afraid to try something else. If you start to slow down, feel helpless, feel like your options are getting narrow or that your world is taking on the same hue as Ann's, seek out some supervisory to help to pull you out of the therapeutic quagmire. Most of all, listen to your inner voice and teach your client to do the same; respect your intuitions, trust your and the client's creativity.

Looking Within: Chapter 15 Exercises

1. What are your reactions to, your values regarding the notion of helping others become change-agents? When is it therapeutic and when manipulative? How do you know?

2. What are your own countertransference issues when working with individuals? What specific emotional dangers could undermine the therapy you are seeking to provide? How do you resolve for yourself the issue of the therapeutic relationship as the primary arena for change versus changes accomplished with others outside of therapy?

3. Does your focus on the past, on inner dynamics, change when seeing an individual rather than seeing a family? Why or why not?

4. Imagine your intimate partner were to come to your individual therapy to present his or her view of a major problem between you both. How do you think you would react? How might it help or hinder your solving of the problem, your relationship? How do you feel about bringing in others to the sessions as consultants? What would make you hesitate about doing this?

[16]

Staying Sane

SURVIVAL TIPS FOR THERAPISTS

One of the goals of this book has been to show you how to apply some of the basic assumptions and principles of family therapy. The other has been to encourage your creative thinking, to help you see that there are many therapeutic roads to the same end. If you can be clear about your goals, flexible in your approach, pragmatic in your philosophy—and have the humility to make mistakes and the courage to fly by the seat of your pants—you can be effective in your clinical practice.

Fine, you say, but how do you do this over the long haul? How do you stay creative in the face of endless tales of abuse, despair, chaos, frustration? How do you stay sane and committed, rather than numb, bitter, cynical, or even hostile?

The answer, of course, is that you need to treat yourself the way you treat your clients, namely, to push yourself out of your comfort zone and against your grain just as the family members have to push themselves in order to make changes in themselves, their families, their world. Once again, the therapeutic buck stops with you. But that also doesn't mean you grind it out all alone. Like your families, you can get help and support along the way.

In this chapter, a catalogue of sorts, we'll consider the idea of self-care for the family therapist: ways to keep your creative juices flowing and your options open, ways to stay grounded and sensitive without becoming emotionally overwhelmed. We're talking about doing for yourself what you want your families to learn to do for themselves.

STAND BY ME:
THE SUPERVISOR–CONSULTANT CONNECTION

Clients come to you for help with their children, their marriage, themselves. You go to your supervisor for help with the assessment, to develop strategies, to help you become less emotionally entangled. The parallel is obvious. A good supervisor or consultant isn't there to solve your personal problems, but like a good therapist, is there as a support, a parent, a teacher, a sounding board, a brainstormer, a coach, a cheerleader, a storyteller, a friend; he or she is there to push you or pull you up when you need it. Just like a therapist, the supervisor's individual personality is less important than how he or she interacts with you. It's not the person, after all, that helps us to change and grow, but the relationship that we both create together.

The best kind of supervisors are those who have skills and knowledge that you lack. But they are also more than walking textbooks or catalogues of therapeutic skills. The good supervisor not only fills you up with information, but helps you shape that information into a professional self and style that ultimately becomes the very best you.

In order to do this you need a supervisor who appreciates your learning style, whether it be learning by watching your supervisor in action first; planning, preparing, and mapping out your sessions with your supervisor carefully in advance; or jumping right in and asking questions in supervision later. Only by supporting your way of learning, rather than pushing you to follow his or hers, can your supervisor help you develop your own approach, your own voice, your own unique weaving of personality and skill.

A good supervisor also needs to be sensitive to your level of professional development. Learning to do therapy is in many ways like learning to speak a foreign language. Competence is more than the ability to memorize a list of words or clinical interventions; it is measured by an ability to use these tools—to *think* in the language of therapy—and adapt them to a wide range of situations. But this takes time, and moves in stages. The novice, for example, will need more direction and straight-ahead information than someone more advanced; the performance pressure of the beginning may give way to the therapist's true dependence on the supervisor, and this may in turn eventually lead to an adolescent stage of testing, questioning, and separating from the supervisor's own model before the therapist can reach a more integrated self. A good supervisor is flexible. Like a good parent, he or she is able to anticipate your changing needs, is flexible enough to provide the variety of support that you require over time, and is able to change his or her supervisory style and skills to match your own.[1]

This is where good supervision most emulates good therapy. The good supervisor appreciates the organic nature of the relationship. He or she, like the good therapist, knows that it's through the process itself—the negotiating and sorting and solving that goes on between you both—that growth occurs. The supervisor believes that in the development of the relationship between you and him or her comes the development of the professional self within you both.

Like in good therapy, the good supervisor helps you clear out the emotional underbrush that can get in your way of taking risks or being successful. Often it's your anxiety, doubt, anger, or worry that is the main problem with a case. You're anxious about what to do, or what to do right, worried about doing it right, angry that the family isn't changing the way you want them to. The good supervisor helps you sort and sift out these feelings and agendas so you can best use and trust what you already know.

Bad supervision or consultation is the opposite of responsiveness and collaboration. Like bad therapy, bad parenting, and bad marriages, the relationship becomes stale and stifling because both of you are boxed into empty patterns. Rather than developing individuality, the focus is on cloning. Difficult topics are avoided rather than approached. The therapist quickly outgrows the supervisor's rigid learning format, and the supervisor comes to resent the therapist for doing so.

It's your job to make sure you get supervision that both supports and challenges you, that helps you learn and use what you learn. Most of all find someone who gives you the permission and courage to make mistakes, someone who teaches you not only how to correct them but helps you learn the lessons that the mistakes hold.

Of course, there are burned-out or controlling supervisors out there, and you may get routinely assigned to one at your job. If there is a problem, if you feel that the relationship, is not a good fit, if your styles or philosophies are just too vastly different, speak up. Be clear about what you

---

[1]For more information on this developmental approach to clinical supervision, see my book *Clinical Supervision: A Four Stage Process of Growth and Discovery*, Families International, 1995. Copies are available directly from me. I can be reached through The Guilford Press.

want and need, but don't settle. You don't want clients to do that to you, and you needn't do that with your supervisor.

STEPPING BACK: SELF-SUPERVISION

If you think about supervising yourself, more likely than not your mind heads for all that's negative: a mental wagging of a finger at you for being so tough on that mother; the scowling face of your father, your mother, your old mentor scolding you for missing the signs of depression in that father; that small, snarly voice saying "Caught you!" whenever you get offtrack and seem confused.

Some claim that while this harsh, critical-parent image of self-supervision can help keep us on our toes, the self-pummeling can also leave us too cautious and uncreative. Others in the field counter that the danger isn't that we'll be too hard on ourselves, but too easy. The blind spots, rationalizations, and contradictions in what we do are impossible for us to see by ourselves, let alone change. We have no business trying to supervise ourselves. We need someone else, someone not necessarily with wisdom, but with a simple outside perspective to help us see what we're doing.

In between the dangers of being too easy or too hard on ourselves is the view that self-supervision can be a means of reflecting, of stepping back and away from your work in order not to scold but to discover. Following the path of your anxiety and emotions can cast new light on your assumptions. By tracking the patterns of your practice, in much the same way we encourage families to look at the patterns in their own lives, you can recognize the themes that run our living and work.

Sit down with any of your colleagues at lunch one day and listen to each other describe his or her caseload—the problems, the assessment, his or her plan of action. Avoid the temptations of getting swept up in the details of the families' lives or dickering over the right diagnosis, but instead just listen carefully as the stories each tells unfold. Tom, you realize, almost always struggles with resistant fathers "who need to be more responsible"; Nancy sniffs out "fragmentation in the family structure" and is set on getting everyone back and in their proper places; Jamal finds that many of his clients have "suppressed anger" that needs to be expressed in order to increase their personal power; Joy uses a genogram like a road map to invariably track down some "unresolved grief," some "unspoken trauma."

The themes and patterns will begin to stand out before you. The fact that you notice them doesn't make their clinical assessment invalid or the work ineffective. Their impressions are, after all, wrapped around their favorite theories. The pause comes only with curiosity and questioning: Why does that particular theory seems so true to them? Why do all their clients seem to have such consistent underlying problems and needs? What is it that your colleagues see in their families that may tell them what they need? These are the questions that if asked and answered can help keep the projections down; they can keep the therapy from twisting and becoming a vicarious outlet for the therapist's own unexpressed emotions.

What you do and see in your friends you can do for yourself. Take the time to reflect on your own work. What is that treatment plan that you instinctively find yourself writing over and over? What kind of cases or problems are most difficult? How much do your solutions reflect a working on autopilot rather than a carefully tuned, road-tested plan of action? How much are the unique aspects of the family blurred, so that they all conveniently fit into the same few boxes? What is your latest diagnosis of the month? Why?

Taking the time to purposefully reflect in this way helps you slow down and see each family more clearly. Rather than the family turning into the "the two o'clock appointment with the ADHD kid," you have time to sort through your wider impressions and reactions. You have a chance to step back and evaluate how you are responding to everyone in the family, rather than just getting caught up in "getting the parents to set some structure." Small cracks in your approach—for example, your failing to get the father consistently involved—can be noticed and fixed before they develop into something larger, such as, the father starting to undermine the structure.

Such self-reflection is also vital to your creativity. To be creative requires a stirring of the intellectual and emotional pot, so to speak, and then a letting go so that the bits of impressions and images can settle and sit. They can also form new combinations that can produce new insights and approaches. When you cut off this process by shutting off your thoughts at the end of the hour, your work is more likely to reflect your clinical habits and formulas.

Finally, self-reflection helps you recognize your own countertransference. Often your pushing the session out your mind after it's over is a way of pushing away uncomfortable reactions and emotions. By taking the time to dwell on them in a deliberate way, you may discover exactly the problem that's causing you to feel stuck.

How you make time for self-supervision depends upon your working style. Some therapists take time when they are writing up their session notes to look back over the work on the case so far. Others set a time aside each week, an hour perhaps, specifically to reflect upon their entire case-load; make specific time for it at the front end of your weekly planning. Consider a annual, year-end review of your work in order to discern the larger patterns. Read through old cases, remember the ones long gone. What patterns do you see and hear? What common assessment, struggles, goals? What kinds of clients did you seem to hold onto, while others fell away after a few sessions? How flexible was your own style and approach, how rigid? How has your perspective changed now? What developmental issues of yours—breaking away from parents, becoming a parent, establishing your own sense of mastery, dealing with death, becoming a wise man or woman—are reflected in your work, coloring your perspective, changing the shape of your practice, recasting your values?

Tap into your emotions. So you are frustrated with Mr. Jones, angry for some reason at Mrs. Wilson. Go ahead, imagine him sitting there with his arms crossed in front of him, see her with that half-smirk on her face. Tell him what you are thinking; tell her how you feel. Now switch chairs. What would he say back, how would she translate that smirk into words? Switch back again; respond back. Switch again. Notice how the conversation has changed, how you are feeling less frustrated and angry, perhaps, and more depressed or compassionate, how he or she looks less critical and more helpless. Who else from your past or present could you put in the chair that reminds you of these people, this dialogue, these emotions?

Write a brief short story about those clients you're having a hard time with. Use them as characters, making them as dramatic and sympathetic as you can. See what you learn about their motives, their dreams. Put yourself and therapy in the story. What can the fictional process tell you about the real one?

You're sorting out your countertransference, you're owning your projections, you're separating out you from the family. Use those lagging emotions, that afterburn following a session, to discover something about you and them. Self-supervision can help you recharge yourself and the therapy.

TRAINING AND EDUCATION

Want to learn how to work with sexually abused children? Trying to integrate psychodrama into your group work? Need new techniques for working with violent teens? Interested in learning how to apply mindfulness to couple therapy? Then get yourself to a conference or workshop. Get yourself some training.

Short-term training opportunities obviously help you increase your skills, keep you on top of the latest and maybe greatest developments in the field. They also provide those invaluable side benefits of getting you out of the office, taking you to a city where you haven't been before, giving you a chance to meet and re-meet colleagues that you would probably never see otherwise. When you are feeling burned out or discouraged, short trainings can recharge you by helping you see that there is more that you can do, that there are ways to overcome the places in your practice where you feel the most stuck. Sitting in a room with hundreds or thousands of other therapists validates not only that you are not the only one struggling, but also that you in fact belong to a larger therapy family.

Should you desire to delve even deeper into any subject, there is always the extended trainings—the three-week, one month variety, the online course. Rather than just a taste of a particular skill or approach, you can get a whole meal. Beyond that is the intensive, ongoing training, usually leading to some certification—the two-year program in hypnosis, Imago, or Internal Family Systems, the three-year investigation of object relations. Not only is your commitment of time and money obviously greater, but also is the commitment to that approach. You need to be clear about your objectives: What is it that you most want to learn? Why now? How does it fit or conflict with your values? How does it fit with your internal image of whom you want to be?

The questions are important because the answers, which on the surface seem so transparent, quickly turn murky with a bit of reflection. If, for example, you are burned out on what you are doing, or are at that stage of development that you are beginning to outgrow your supervision and are feeling restless, the impression that you want something else, something more—increased energy, a new perspective that cuts through your hodgepodge of techniques—may be strong, but undefined. It's tempting to grasp onto something that at least points a direction, some release from the tension or depression that you feel.

The program may do just that—catch you up in something that's new, that gives you a new way of defining yourself and what you do. But it also may be a mistake if you're not honest with yourself about what you are really seeking and feeling. The restlessness or burnout may merely be a symptom of a larger problem and not the problem itself.

Often the best course is to wait, rather than jumping in, to sit through the transition period and see what happens, rather than becoming impatient and grasping onto something just to have it to hold onto. You may discover that the problem has nothing to do with your professional practice and more to do with your personal needs.

Once you've clarified your clinical needs and goals, however, these extended training sessions can indeed help you feel more grounded, solid, and expert in your work. In contrast to a conference or workshop that gives you new ideas or techniques to supplement your work, immersion in the more intensive training format can literally transform it.

Like good supervision, long-term training should challenge you to discover a deeper level of yourself than short-term training usually does. At its best, extended training shouldn't only give you a few more details about what you already know, or reconfirm what you already believe, but push you to look at what you're doing with fresh eyes, help you to see yourself in a new context and discover what makes you tick. In fact any good, rigorous course of study, even if it is outside your field—literature, mathematics, music, rock climbing—can be worthwhile if you come away from it intellectually and emotionally stretched.

TEACHING

The learning process can be divided up into four stages: (1) You know what you don't know; (2) you don't know what you know; (3) you don't know what you don't know; (4) you know what you know.

In the first stage, as a beginner, you're filled with anxiety because you're only aware of your incompetence, what you don't know. Much of what you do feels like you're barely keeping your head above water. You mistakenly believe that others see your incompetence as well and are not mentioning it only in order to be polite.

In the second, you've gained ground, you've learned more, but pieces of what you've learned remained scattered in your mind—you don't know what you know. You haven't been able to bring them together to give yourself a solid framework from which to practice. Instead, you often wind up winging it—pulling out bits of theory here, samples of techniques there—and feeling once again like a beginner.

In the third stage your knowledge and skills consolidate and your sense of confidence and power grows. In fact, like an adolescent, you're aware only of your power and you see only what you know—your way is the best way. You feel on top of things, but in this haughty frame of mind you don't realize the limits of your knowledge and experience—you don't know what you don't know. Your vision is myopic; you're often not aware of the subtleties of your approach; you can easily ignore the larger implications and effects of what you're doing. Your sense of self-importance, your uncritical loyalty to your beliefs, may make you may take unnecessary risks.

In the final stage you come back down to earth; you're more humble about your skills and knowledge. Like everyone else you have your own strengths and weaknesses—you know what you know, but you're less cocky, more flexible. There isn't one way, you realize, but many. There's always more to learn, but you also know you can trust the foundation of knowledge and skill that you have worked hard to acquire.

In all of these stages the challenge is in defining and using what you know and believe and honestly admitting what you don't. But there's more to this than simply glancing over your shoulder and tallying up what you have and what you don't. Learning to be a therapist involves bringing together all the aspects of who you are. It's an ongoing, developmental climb of building up and peeling away, of supporting and confronting, of giving yourself the break and looking at yourself squarely in the eye.

One useful way of clarifying what you know and what you don't, of uncovering the gaps in your knowledge is through teaching, formally (the classroom, the seminar, the short course, the writing of a journal article) or informally (the brown bag lunch topic, the two-hour staff development for colleagues, the taking on of a student in supervision). Teaching forces you to consolidate your bits of knowledge, to pinpoint and name your hunches and intuitions, and to shape them both into something more integrated, more substantial. In the process of sorting through for others what is important to learn, you have to sort through for yourself what you already know.

The teaching process is also a great antidote to the feeling that you're intellectually treading water. It's easy to become dulled by your own practice, to feel that you "just do what you do." You need the opportunity to rediscover your uniqueness, to reconfirm for others and yourself that what you do works, that your approach represents a unique blend of personality and skills. Teaching, and the feedback that others give about what you say, can do this.

So arrange to have a regular staff development time where each therapist presents his or her own unique approach to helping families. Think about a case or technique that was particularly successful and expand upon its implications. Do a literature review, define your own unique perspective or application and write it up for a journal. Contact your local university and see if you can serve as a field instructor for graduate students in social work, or clinical or counseling psychology. See if they need adjunct teachers. Offer to teach a course on marriage and family at the local community college, or one on parenting through the county continuing adult education program. Make up a flyer of the topics and workshops that you can teach and mail them out to all the Departments of Social Services and Family Courts in your state. You may be surprised by how much you have to offer.

THE QUICK AND EASY: MISCELLANEOUS SURVIVAL SKILLS

Finally there are everyday antidotes to therapy's wear and tear. Here are a few:

• *Diversify.* A caseload filled with 20 hyperactive eight-year-old boys may help you refine your skills, but may also drive you insane. If at all possible, diversify your caseload—a mix of families, problems, personalities; a stable of core cases, perhaps, of what you do best, one or two cases that lead you to learn something new. Create a mix in your daily schedule— seeing four depressed clients in a row on a rainy Wednesday afternoon is going to leave you feeling dull and empty. Put a couple of those hyperactive kids in the middle of it all, see a couple after doing some play therapy, an individual adult after three teenagers. If your clients start to sound the same, you'll start to react the same.

Don't be afraid to diversify your work responsibilities as well. Talk to your supervisor about taking part in a community assessment or treatment team, help with agency public relations and marketing, do follow-up research on your clients' satisfaction. These additional activities can break up the grind of doing back-to-back therapy and can give you another perspective on work.

• *Control your time.* This is relatively easy to do in private practice, though, of course, even here how you spend some of your time is going to be determined by client demand. In agency work, however, where others may schedule your appointments, you could wind up with the most chaotic family at the time of day when you are most sluggish and least able to manage them. You know how the case flow over the course of the day affects you, you know when you are at your best, when you need a break to regroup. Set your own schedule.

• *Be proactive about what scares you.* Do you walk around with the dread that you too could get subpoenaed and wind up having to testify in court? Do you worry that the retired gentleman you just started seeing could easily turn actively suicidal and make you feel panicked and helpless? Do you wake up at two in the morning wondering if one of the client's in your anger management group is actually getting too excited and possibly explosive right there in the room?

Everyone has some fear about something that he or she has never yet encountered but eventually could. The dread comes from worrying that this shoe could drop at any time, and, most likely, you imagine, when you're unprepared to handle it.

So spare yourself the worry by preparing yourself for the worst. Talk to your supervisor now about protocols for dealing with subpoenas. Follow one of your more experienced colleagues to court to see what happens and how he or she manages those situations. Sign up for a suicide prevention training or intervention skill training for managing aggressive or violent clients. Be proactive so you can be confident.

• *Allow yourself to relax in sessions.* Beginning therapists often feel that they have to be hypervigilant with clients—never breaking eye contact, constantly making those cow eyes and appropriate sighs and nods of the head to let the client know they are listening. Usually this is attention overkill. Some of the best therapist allow themselves to relax, to stare off into the space just above the client's head. It can be a huge relief and it helps you to listen and think better.

• *Make an effort to spend time with colleagues.* Therapy is isolating. Offset this by scheduling a regular time to have lunch with a colleague up-stairs, have a weekly meeting with everyone in the practice every Thurs-day morning just to check in and touch base, have an informal supervi-sion lunch meeting with a group of practitioners whose work you respect on Wednesdays twice a month.

• *Make your work space as comfortable as possible.* Is that rickety chair driving you crazy? What about the drawer that always sticks, the bland beige walls, the couch with the dark stain and the sagging cushions that you feel embarrassed about every time a new client sits down on it? You spend a good amount of your time in one place—try to make it your own.

Try to make it attractive as well. Take a look at the offices of friends and colleagues to give you creative ideas. How about a nice picture on the wall that reflects your personality or the mood you want to create (skip that painting of Pickett's Charge). Get a small aquarium and a few fish. Shut off the overhead florescent lights and get some attractive lamps. Put down carpeting, or throw down a small oriental-looking rug over the gray-ish, industrial carpeting that's there. Set up the toys on a bookcase rather than heaping them in a cardboard box. Bring in some plants, even fake ones, to help the place look less sterile. Use your imagination. Make it look more like home and less like an office.

• *Do something that helps you feel centered.* Because therapy so easily pulls you into other's lives, it important to have something in your life that can pull you back out, that helps you feel centered, that activates an-other portion of yourself. Meditation twice a day, running, cooking din-ner, playing the piano, writing a novel, rafting, gardening, singing—whatever it is, find something that puts you somewhere else (preferably legal and not addicting), that lets you drop the day's events from your mind, that makes you feel competent, healthy, powerful, or positive about who you are and what you do.

• *Take vacations.* Not working vacations, but real vacations that help you either relax and stimulate you, but certainly are different than your everyday life. Go to the beach for a week and bring novels, not journals. Go to Pennsylvania, but instead of going to see your mother or Aunt

Rosie, stay in Philadelphia and take in the sights. Or go see your mother and Aunt Rosie, but stop off in Philadelphia anyhow.

• *Have a balanced personal life.* Easier said than done, of course. But if you want to avoid the dangers we have been talking about—the vicarious acting out through your clients, the need for their intimacy, all the ways that therapy can be distorted because you have come to personally need more from it than the rest of your life provides—you need to discover and stay involved in the rest of your life. If you need doing therapy more than your clients need the therapy, everyone is in trouble.

• *Have realistic expectations.* Like any other craft or art it takes time— eight to 10 years is probably reasonable—to hone your skills and style, to begin to master the subtleties of practice, to feel confident in what you do. Some therapists, often the most sensitive ones it seems, give up too quickly. They get so frustrated and critical of themselves in those early years over what they're aware that they don't know, that they leave the field before they have a chance to develop their skills and get really good. Be patient with yourself and don't box yourself in with unrealistic expectations.

These survival skills, along with good supervision, training, and opportunities to teach what you know can help you stay sane, stable, and even steadily enthusiastic about your work over the long haul. The overriding theme here is one of balance and diversity—of putting your emotional eggs in several baskets so that you don't have to clutch too tightly to just one, finding many ways of expressing yourself, of working, of discovering what lies within.

Finally, it's also important to find balance in your therapeutic role. One of the important and often subtle shifts that I see good therapists make as they gain experience is in seeing their responsibility less as fixing the presenting problem that the family brings in and more as helping the family fix it themselves. Therapy and the therapist don't solve the problem, but instead provide a forum for doing so. The therapist can help the family understand how and why the problem came about, point out what they're doing to each other and themselves and speculate on how it might be connected to their concerns, give them a place and way of talking about ideas and options, and support them in what they decide to do. But what they ultimately do is up to them, not you, the therapist. As the first chapter pointed out, therapy is only one way of approaching problems. Your sanity and satisfaction, and that of your clients as well, comes in accepting and appreciating your limits.

Looking Within: Chapter 16 Exercises

1. How do you learn best? What do you need most from supervision or consultation? How have your needs changed over the past year? What would be most difficult to talk about in supervision? Why? How can you repair/expand that relationship? Change it to better meet your clinical need and personal needs? How can you make time for self-supervision of your work?

2. List all the reasons you give yourself for not taking advantage of some kind of extended training. How much would it be worth to feel 50% more competent as a therapist? How can you overcome the obstacles?

3. What can you teach? What can't you teach but would like to? What's stopping you? Make a list of all the possible teaching opportunities in your area.

4. How can you change your work environment—physically, socially, emotionally—to make it less stressful?

5. Be honest—how's your personal life? How is it affecting your work life? What can you do to change it?

[17]

The Lessons of Therapy

Therapy is a way of thinking. What you do isn't as important as how you think about what you do. You sort and shift, finding one fact to be more important than another, one sigh meaning more than whatever is being said. You organize all that you hear and see into a picture that you then hand back to the family. This is what I see, you say. They pass the picture around and turn it this way and that. They tell you that you've made them look funny, or misshapen, or have left out something important, or they are startled or relieved by what they see. The accuracy of the picture is less important than the opportunity it provides for the family to begin to think about themselves in a new way.

Therapy is an approach to life. Even before anything is said in the office, before the client makes that first phone call to you, there's a shared belief that problems and relationships can change only with the support of others. Living, we agree, isn't a solo act, rarely smooth and easy. It's a bumpy road where we fall and skin our knees and where we sometimes get lost. But by talking about what is painful, confusing, frustrating, depressing, even with strangers, it can become less so. We need others to help us get up, to point the way, to walk beside us.

We—you and I—started this exploration of family therapy by stepping back and looking at its assumptions and foundations. In this chapter we swing back around and look once again at this thing we call therapy, but with a wider perspective of our own personal work lives and everyday living.

Specifically, we'll be looking for and at those places where what you do and what you believe clash, where your values are trodden on by the pace and pattern of your everyday life, where what you do and what you feel are disjointed. It is here, in the neglect, contradiction, and disparity of your practice that the seams and eventually the structure of your work and life are most likely to weaken and your professional and personal self can drift off course. It is here where you suddenly find that the distance between who you are and what you do has become wide indeed.

As we move through this chapter, try to step back and look at your work life in its entirety, become curious about the way and how well therapy and your work represents the larger self that is you. Look for the gaps, the places where important parts of yourself are ignored or where your self-honesty is clouded by rationalizations and routine.

THERAPY AS TEACHER

The lens of therapy is capable of focusing upon the smallest, most elemental, concentrated forms of our psychological lives. But what do we see when we look? Some ideas:

• *It's not individuals who help us to heal, but relationships with those individuals.* We talked about this from the beginning, and saw this validated in the stories of Billy, the boy traumatized by the murder of his brother, and Ellen, the teenager struggling to replace her deceased father. It's not the rider or the horse that wins the race, but both working together; it's not you fixing someone, nor the family necessarily fixing themselves. Whatever positive or negative that happens in the session happens in the present within the smallest of psychic spaces between you and them. It is this therapeutic alchemy, the mixing together of elements from each other's worldview and living, that makes something new.

But what are the desirable qualities of those relationships? Reliability—not missing sessions or being late; following though on promises made, offers accepted. Being present, giving over the entire time to being concerned about the client. To care about them, not for our sake, but theirs. To care about and take responsibility for what happens in the session but not to care too much or take responsibility for what happens outside of it. To accept differences but to look for commonalities. To have integrity in that your words and behaviors in the moment represent, as much as you are able, your true thoughts and feelings. To be as absolutely honest as you can be.

• *We constantly re-create our past.* From each new vantage point in the present we look back on our past and see it anew. As the research on trauma and false memory suggests, our past is not the granite-like foundation on which we build our present and personality; instead it is a shadowy and fragile thing always connected to our present. The start of a new job reminds us of past other beginnings, and we both feel again those feelings of excitement and worry, as well as look at those times in a different way. A loss—divorce, death of a parent or friend—brings to mind other losses and other deaths, and we mentally comb through them, uncovering patterns of regret and resolutions that we didn't notice before. Our losses, we discover, shape us more than our successes, our failures are prerequisites for our growth.

Our present, past, and in turn our future are fluid and interconnected. As therapists we make use of this interrelationship in our work. By helping to create changes on one dimension of time—for example, by asking everyone about good memories of the past—we stimulate change in the present and future.

• *Symptoms and problems are interchangeable perspectives.* When have we really reached the core problem? When are presenting issues the center of our focus and when are they just smoke and dust, distracting us and the family from what lies beyond? When is a problem not really a problem but a mere symptom of a something larger, less defined?

The fluidity of time is mirrored in the fluidity of problems and symptoms and shaped by the eyes of the beholder. What we call problems are our attempts to capture and name for a moment the emotions, memories, and needs flowing within, which are too difficult to name and hold. The name is less important than the process of naming. When we hand our picture back to the family our purpose is not to shake them and make them see once and for all the Problem that's right there in front of their faces; rather, we're opening the door and inviting them to step into the pool of memory and emotion from which the problem comes.

• *Life is made up of patterns.* Once we step into process that makes up the problem, we and they can see the patterns that compose it. It's these patterns that we map and follow in sessions with our clients.

But the patterns are us, the therapists, as well. Like our clients, we too created our own patterns long ago as children, to survive. They can keep our lives stable, but they can also become outdated and no longer represent who we truly are. They can become ineffective and limit our power as therapists.

If I learned, for example, to accommodate rather than confront people who seem to intimidate me, both my feeling of intimidation and my fear of their reaction to my challenge are based upon childhood fears that in effect keep me a child. So I hold back at times in my personal life, falling into habits and responses that help me feel safe, but often resentful. When I do the same in therapy I risk replicating the dysfunctional process in the family, overidentifying with the victim or inadvertently encouraging someone else in the family to fight my battle. I am less powerful, less able to put what I know into practice, less a good role model. We need to be able to confront and change the patterns that make up our lives as we internally change.

• *Self-awareness is the ability to step out of the patterns, to adopt a different perspective.* There is a Chinese proverb that says, "There is no shame in growing slowly, only in standing still." Many of the families that we see feel they have little control over their lives because they are standing still as life swirls around them. Our job in the therapeutic process is to offer our view as an outsider—a different look at the relationship, a new slant on the past. The newness of what they see through your eyes can help pull the family out of the stuckness of their current life and get them moving toward higher ground. From this different place not only can they catch their breath, but they can see the flow of the current that was carrying them. These become the "Aha" experiences of therapy.

You and I need to be able to do the same—to step outside our own lives from time to time in order to get away from the craziness we may feel by seeing the bigger picture and our place. We need to take the time to reflect on the routines and rules that we automatically follow and see if they still fit. We need to question the vision that we hold of our lives and be willing to change it. We need to move about mentally and emotionally and move toward the unknown so that we don't lose the capacity or create the fear within us of moving at all.

It is in the movement within the moment, with risk, action, and honesty where relationships live, where our life visions are created, where the stepping back occurs, where the anxiety is felt. The content is always secondary to the process, the moving toward is more important than the arriving.

These are some of the notions that I see woven in the therapy process. You may discover others. The purpose of asking what therapy teaches you about life is not about discovering truth, but merely once again helping you to define the values and assumptions hidden within your work and to encourage you build your work and life on the same foundation.

LIFE AS WORK

This unity of life and work is what we most often associate with the artist: for example, Mary Cassatt struggling to capture on the canvas the vision that fills her brain; Mozart and Beethoven, driven to translate the feelings inside in notes on a page so that others may hear the sounds and experience the emotions; Virginia Woolf, who dedicates five years of her life to create the perfect novel, one that carries the reader so completely into the world that she alone creates within her mind. We're drawn to this way of life not only because it seems so unstructured compared to the nine-to-five routine into which most of us feel wedged, but mostly because it seems so *committed*, so *creative*.

This is work that flows from the inside out, rather than from the outside in, work that soaks in all of who and what you are. It is work that goes beyond the boundaries of a "good job" with its means to other ends, or the "career," that track that we follow to some ultimate level or publicly recognized success. This is work as a calling.

While the notion of a calling conjures up the sound of celestial choirs and beams of radiant light falling down on you from above, it most often begins with only a whisper of some inner voice telling you that this is something you should do, the flicker of an image across your mind that gradually, over time, grows into a vision that pulls you forward. A calling is realized when you step back from what you are already doing and sense that this work is something that you are not only good at, but were meant to do. You have found a medium for expressing who you most are. Like the artist, you become caught up in the flow of the work, you can lose sense of time, you are absolutely engaged. You do the work not because of what you might get for it at some time in the future, but because of what the doing does for you in the present.

So what is that calling for you? Why do you do therapy or want to do therapy? What does it offer you as a medium? How does actualize your values and beliefs, your sense of purpose and creativity? Why do you need to do it?

If you are not sure that therapy is your calling, then what is? What is it that you can't wait to do when you wake up in the morning? What do the dreams, the visions, the fantasies that you have tell you about what you need to do most?

I'm aware that we're not talking about everyday practicality or reality. Sure, you need to have a job for money, to have a place to live, to send your kids to college, to survive in the real world. But unless you have the courage to periodically ask these bigger questions, the gap between your work and yourself will gradually widen. You will feel cynical, tired, and burned out—frustrated and fed up. You will find yourself one day in the middle of a 20-, or 30-, or 40-year crisis, filled with fantasies and ready to run away toward dreams that have only become more desperate and powerful by your neglect. If you don't build your work around your life, you can easily wind up building your life around your work.

LIFE OF INTEGRITY

Actually, "building" may be the wrong word. Do we really build our lives? Many would say yes, especially considering the society we live in. Images of American pioneers, those self-sufficient, hard-working, brave frontiersmen and -women who created their lives out of nothing more than hope and sweat and guts are incorporated within each of us. We have, we're told, roughly 40 years—from 20 to 60 years old—to do the same, to grab hold of our lives in our two hands and make something out of it. At the end of the time you and everyone else will take stock and look at just how much you've accomplished, how well you have done, how successful you are.

But there is another point of view, another way of looking at our relationship to living. Rather than building our lives we discover them. This is the notion of a life unfolding, the sense that our lives are led, the image of it staying always a few steps ahead of us, around the corner, gently waving its hand, urging us to follow. It's an image that tells us that by staying close to ourselves, with our ear pressed tight against the ground of our lives, listening—to our intuitions, our emotions, our fantasies—we will discover our purpose, our calling. We will live the life we were meant to have.

The split between these two perspectives is like that of context and process; they are two sides of the same reality. Building at its worst becomes a left-brain-driven forced march to success and accomplishment. Discovery at its worst lacks grounding; weightless visions and fragile dreams float forever within our heads but never enter our lives. The best is the combination of both, where discovery becomes the thin lines on a sheet of blueprint paper and building becomes the nailing of rafters and beams into the solid structure that we call our life.

Both are important, but like its sister, process, it is discovery that leads the way. To give credence and respect to this side of our lives is only to do what we do with our families—helping them to give full voice to whispers and nods, helping them to step aside for a moment from the pain that their problem may be creating in order to hear what their problem is telling them about what they need to learn, asking those "miracle questions" to help them draw out the answers within them that they didn't know were there. Even when they feel victimized and battered by life, we say to them that life, their life, is ready to give something back to them if only they have the courage to open their eyes and live it.

When we scrape down to the bottom of this way of thinking, we find ourselves resting once again on assumption, values, even faith—a faith that we can not only find our purpose, but that there is purpose; that problems not only have solutions, but lessons to teach us; and that once we learn the lessons, the problems miraculously disappear. This is not the calm, sedentary faith that reassures us that everything will turn out all right, but the wild, robust faith that comes from living by the seat of our pants.

If you are able to live this way, to wait and listen, then go to work to make your inner and outer life mirror to each other, then your life is filled with gut-sure honesty, with true integrity. It will be a different life than the carefully built one that keeps discovery locked away, that sets its marker early on and moves steadily forward. To bring faith and discovery and honesty into your life, into your work, is to walk out on a trail on a crisp morning following the sound of the hawk flying above rather than the painted sign on the tree. You may suddenly you find yourself sitting out on a limb or looking over the edge of a cliff and not know why or how you got there. You may look down and feel afraid, but if you look inside you will find courage; if you look up, you will see visions.

Looking Within: Chapter 17 Exercises

1. Draw a picture of your life. Get crayons, pencils, paint, and a large sheet of paper, and write at the top "My Life." Let your unconscious lead you—follow the images that come to mind, the memories that may be stirred up, the feelings that you have. Give yourself about 15 minutes. Then let the picture sit for a day, then look at it carefully again.

2. What do your recurring problems tell you about what you need to learn? How can doing therapy, or your clients themselves, help you learn those lessons?

3. How do you look back on your past different now than you did five or 10 years ago? How has this image changed your sense of the present, the future?

4. What did you want to be when you grew up? How have you incorporated those characteristics into your current work?

5. How close is the gap between your inner and outer world? What would it take to bring them together?

Index